FITTER.
CALMER.
STRONGER.

ELLIE GOULDING

SEVEN DIALS

To all the brilliant, resilient women in my life and beyond, Caspar, and my little Arthur . . .

CONTENTS

Introduction

I'm not even going to try and play it cool: I'm really excited that you've picked up this book (or decided to listen to the audio version). Either way, thank you for investing your precious time into learning more about my approach to health and fitness.

This is a book I've been secretly passionate about writing for a while. In truth, exercise and fitness have long played an incredibly important role in my life. (This is not to say I've always got it right, as we shall discover.) I've had a pretty colourful life so far, mostly because of where my joy for music and singing has taken me, and I have experienced all manner of ups and downs. But through everything, when I really think about it, the one constant that has never let me down is training. My exercise and my strength have proved to be the two things I have always managed to maintain, even when times have been particularly testing. When I've felt totally overwhelmed, I've been able to use my movement as a consistent way of getting through tough times.

My voice, my music and writing will always be my mysterious, unpredictable, fiery friend for life. But even if I write something I love, I can't always rely on it to make me feel good. The truth is I often write my best songs when I'm feeling miserable.

So a couple of years ago I began to wonder if I could, in a sense, even out the highs and lows and – as training has been such an incredible companion to me – could I up the ante? Could I really integrate fitness and wellbeing so that my health story (we all have one of these) could underpin everything I did?

Now, this didn't mean that I intended to swap the studio and dedicate myself to becoming a professional athlete. I wasn't going to give up music to become a boxer (although honestly I love boxing so much, I think my manager sometimes worries this might be on the cards). My husband, Caspar, is from the world of elite athletics – he's a rower. And as much as I've learned from his mindset and experiences (it's very useful to share your life with an athlete when you want training tips), our respective approaches differ wildly. Whereas I want to use my training and up my knowledge about my body and wellbeing to prepare myself to be a fitter and stronger person in any situation, Caspar's objective is usually to win!

You'll notice I often refer to 'training', rather than 'working out', because I believe when you move your body, you are training yourself physically and mentally for whatever lies ahead of you in life. A common question I get asked is 'What are you training for?' And I'll say, 'Well, just life.' It helps me remember that moving my body isn't a punishment for anything, or to compensate for any slip ups, but to help me remember just how alive I can feel.

When I began to make breakthroughs in my own training and feel a transition in my mental health and make that all-important connection between the two (which we'll talk about a lot, particularly in Chapter 3, 'Calm Your Mind'), I began to get really excited about sharing my experience more formally. I began quietly wondering if I could turn what I'd learned into a programme that you could follow. And at some point my quiet intentions got blurted out (perhaps after a few wines) and, well, here we are – it's happening!

Throughout this book I'll use my life and experiences to explain how I've arrived at my conclusions. I'm going to do this, because it would be super-weird if I didn't mention what I've been up to for the last thirty-four years. I also think that there are lessons to be found not just in the stuff that happened, but often in my reactions. (You can thank me later by the way for refraining from referring to these as 'teachable moments', which makes me feel a bit ill.) I think to know our bodies and how they work in a really useful way, we have to examine not just what we've navigated, but how we react at the time. But

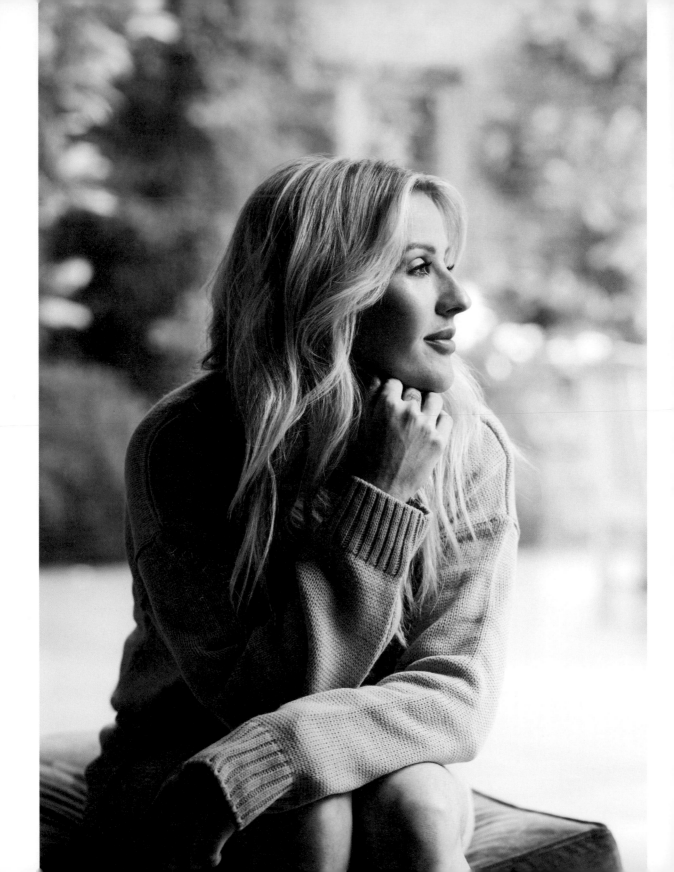

I don't want you to worry: this is definitely not a book about being a fabulous pop star and how we're completely unique and very special people. Erm, because we're not. The problems and barriers that stop us achieving our fitness and health potential are ones that we've all come across. The themes I'll tackle are universal.

But this book will feel a bit different from many other fitness plans. (And that's deliberate, not because we forgot to do it properly.) So nowhere in this book will you find any mentions of baby weight, a twenty-eight-day plan or a promise to drop a stone or a dress size, or an instruction to cut anything out. You won't find those instructions because THEY DON'T REALLY WORK! At least not in the long term, and not for me. And they definitely don't make you happy. Health and fitness is so much more complex than a twenty-eight-day plan or attaining a goal weight.

Instead, in this book you'll find lots of kind, encouraging and, I hope, very helpful advice about how to navigate your own health and find your brightest self. I see this book as a manual, a set of principles and a source for anyone who wants to dip in. I'd love for it to be something you can rely on. I like to imagine you'll get to know it really well, and dip in when you need to correct your course in life or need some inspiration or support. I'd love you to really use it – folding over the corners of a couple of your favourite pages, or underlining sentences that particularly chime. When it comes to the routines and programmes put together by our stellar experts, we've gone for an old-school format of written down instructions. Personally, I love a low-tech approach – I love a training programme that I can carry with me (without having to remember to charge my iPad) and one where I can even write my own notes in the margins. But please do not do this if you are borrowing this book from a mate. And if you're reading in a bookshop, hoping to find your brightest self for free – then, fine . . . but do buy the copy after!

This is a book you'll want to own, not least for the incredible experts who have contributed in the following chapters. There's my friend Fearne Cotton, who I've known since the start of my career, and who you'll find being characteristically brilliant in Chapter 3, 'Calm Your Mind', as she explains how looking after her emotional health has gone from being something she found daunting to one of her favourite things to do. In Chapter 4, 'Nourish Your Body', the amazing nutritionist Pixie Turner reveals how to eat well without overcomplicating things. In Chapter 5, 'Reset Your Mindset', we'll discuss mindset and learned behaviours with Dr Tamsin Lewis, who combines being a triathlete with neuroscience (I know, what an overachiever!). Then from Chapter 7, 'How I move: the workouts', I hand over to some genuine legends of sport and fitness. Matt Roberts is my personal trainer, and he's going to talk you through five home-based workouts he's designed, each tailored to a different time of day or energy level. Darren Barker is my boxing coach, and his box-fit workout is the same one his dad did to get fit before boxing matches in the 1970s (I think of it as the fitness equivalent to getting my hands on the secret family recipe for a tomato sauce in an Italian family). The champion boxer Katie Taylor will explain how boxing can improve your emotional strength as well as physical fitness. And we finish with Catie Miller, my exceptional barre teacher, taking you through a full-body barre warm-up and sculpt class (a workout inspired by ballet, yoga and Pilates).

I'm incredibly privileged to know these outstanding humans. In fact, it's no exaggeration to say meeting them as friends and professionals has changed the course of my life. I've never really been into team sports, but in many ways they are my team. And now, by extension, they're on your team, too. I'd say that's a win for both of us!

Don't worry if you don't pick up every point, or if you gravitate more to one part of the book than others (being a total geek, I really like the bits on how you can harvest your data and track your performance). We're all about the long term, about how you integrate new habits to underpin your training and help you realise your brightest self (a concept I'll go into in more detail in the next chapter).

In many ways, I see this moment we're living right now as the perfect time to start this transformation. So much about instilling a healthy life that builds resilience is actually about being flexible and adaptable. You know that saying 'roll with the punches'? This is something we've all had to do in our recent past as we were forced to confront the reality of life during a global pandemic. Trying to keep an iron grip on our daily lives suddenly didn't work. In order to keep our routines, we had to adapt. On a practical level, you may have had to change your training to Zoom sessions with friends in living-room workouts or grabbing a moment amid never-ending home-schooling. It was tough, wasn't it? But you made it work and that should give you confidence that you can move through life with both agility and focus.

Of course, the story doesn't end there. Caspar and I decided to push the unpredictability idea a little further. Apparently the global pandemic wasn't enough! By the autumn of 2020 my bid to be fitter, calmer, stronger seemed to be going pretty well. Things were knitting together and my training made me feel if not invincible, at least unstoppable. Then strange things began to happen. Hmmm, I started to feel a little out of breath sometimes. I couldn't quite lift those weights or sustain those reps. I felt so drawn to carbs that I came close to stopping the car if I saw someone eating a sandwich. Daydreaming about milkshakes and fast food, I found it took an extra effort to avoid drive-throughs. A short investigation revealed me to be pregnant.

Pregnancy definitely threw a spanner in my smug self-realisation stage. I was suddenly thrown into the most unpredictable time in my life, with no preparation, completely surrendering myself to the idea that there really was no control, and not necessarily in a fun way that you might get on, say, a night out. My body altered, my hormones went wild and some days I didn't even recognise myself. Not to mention the constant longing for chocolate Weetabix and squirty cream (Pixie Turner, look away now!).

But once Caspar, my friends and I had finished laughing at the irony of it all, I realised this too was an opportunity. Because if you're looking for the ultimate test of things life can throw at you, pregnancy is definitely up there. So while I was confident before that the approach, ideas and format that will unfold over the following chapters can see you through much of what life can throw at you, now I'm 100 per cent convinced. I can safely say I think our plan works because it's been tested in a variety of circumstances including a global pandemic and the safe gestation and delivery of our beautiful baby. So next time someone asks any of us what we're training for, you know the answer. All together now – three, two, one – 'BECAUSE LIFE'!

Shall we begin?

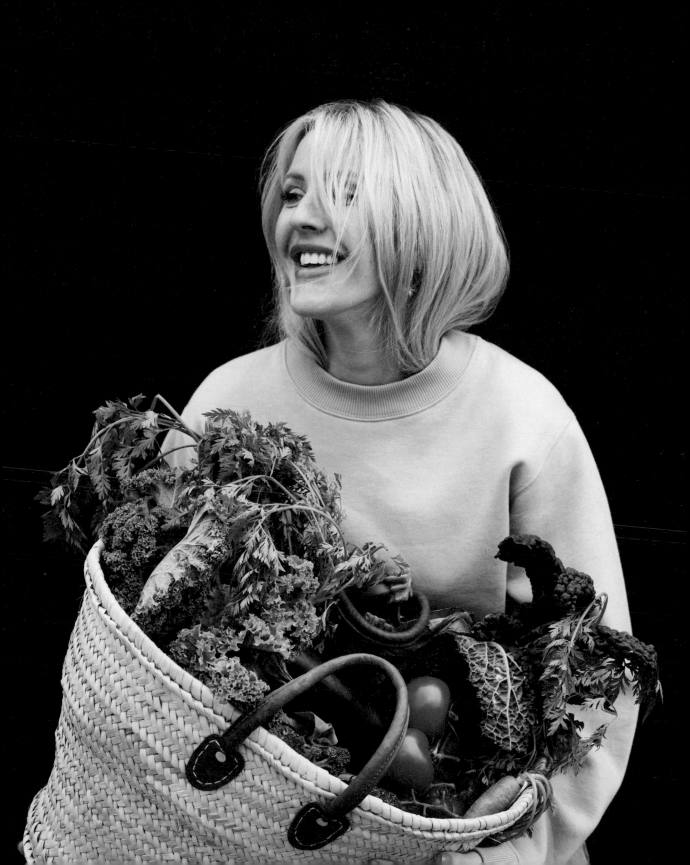

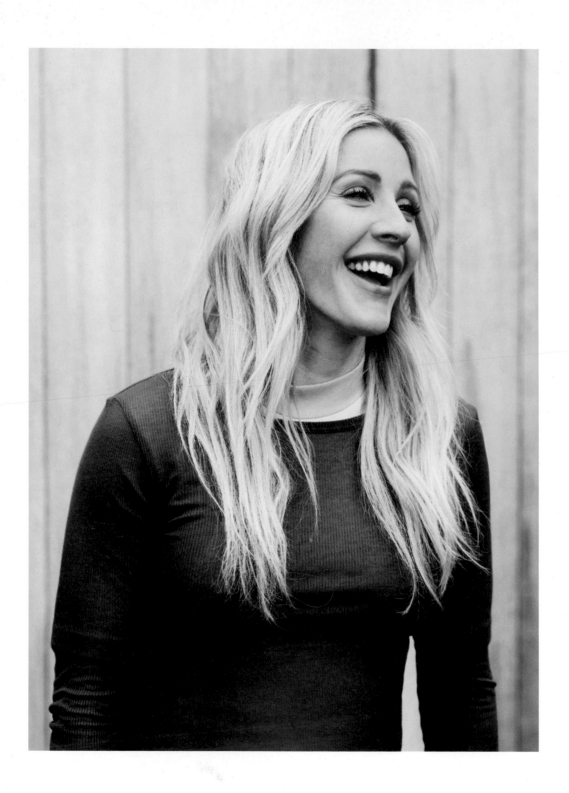

1

BE YOUR BRIGHTEST SELF

'The oak fights the wind, and breaks. The willow bends, and lives on.'

ROBERT JORDAN, AUTHOR

Brightest Self: **a transformation where you aim to be emotionally and physically prepared for the rigours of life. To be empowered, knowing you have the mental agility and strength in your body to be resilient. You can be peaceful when you need peace and have the energy to take off like a rocket when you need to act.**

So many people I know think that fitness and health is about control and rules. No judgement. I mean, I was absolutely convinced it was about those things for a long time! And perhaps staying healthy shouldn't be that complicated, but it becomes loaded – not least with other people's expectations. This has a sort of domino effect. Pressure pushes on fear and fear pushes on perfection. And I know we're all familiar with the latter: honestly, it's like the Perfection Olympics out there – it is madness!

Women in particular have been conditioned to act as if they're competing for the gold medal. But in reality you just run around in a massive circle trying to attain an unattainable standard. 'Have no fear of perfection, you'll never reach it,' said the artist Salvador Dali. I think you'll agree he was definitely on to something, but in practice if you're not a Catalan surrealist painter it can be difficult to disentangle yourself.

Perfectionism often plays out by us seeking control. I've done this for most of life, and you've likely done a lot of it, too. For me, there's a massive misconception when it comes to health and fitness that the more control you assert in order to attain perfection, the more you'll achieve. It kind of makes sense, but it is a trap.

Now you know I didn't come to this realisation overnight. Neither have I ditched all of all my bad habits. I'm definitely a work in progress, but there has been so much progress as I've actively committed to being in charge of my health and improving my diet, my sleep and my training regime. This is a big change. My low days used to be ridiculously low. I just couldn't find a way out of them, and it would set me right back. I often felt as if I was failing because when I felt down I wasn't being productive. Then I'd be preoccupied with silly, irrational thoughts about my life – or rehashing some slight argument I'd had with someone six years beforehand. Finally, I'd forget to move (later in the book, I'll talk about how movement is such a restorative, brilliant thing to do). But honestly I used to forget it was an option! I could quickly set myself up for the shittiest of days.

If you recognise any of this, take a moment to think about how and why you can get caught up in some of these traps. Our personal histories are deeply relevant here.

I work in an industry that has long been associated with recklessness; booze and substances; broken sleep; and constant ups and downs, especially on tour. In short, being a pop star is not associated with balance, sobriety and a big interest in nutrition and total body conditioning. Add on to that the fact that I am from what the media calls a 'normal background', by which they mean a council house in Hereford. From my perspective, I definitely didn't have the most challenging childhood, by which I mean people have had a lot worse. It's just that there were lots of factors in mine, which on their own might have been OK, but all together felt like a lot. My parents got divorced when I was very young, so my dad wasn't a part of my life growing up. And my mum really struggled with money, while having to raise four kids in a small council house. I had a sort of stepfather who I clashed with massively. There was a lot of tension in our house, a lot of stress and a lot of anxiety whirling around between all of us.

All of this means that there was a certain expectation about me, as I think there are with many women in my industry who 'burst' on to the music scene and become successful 'beyond our wildest dreams' – I'm using these phrases because this is the way our story is often written. (By the way, my wild dreams have nothing to do with success!) Of course there have been some crazy moments, and at times I did feel I'd been in the fast spin cycle of a washing machine. But that can be true of any industry. You may well have experienced periods that felt a bit chaotic, where you lost sense of your self and your wellbeing went out the window. It's easily done!

But what I've always felt is that there was a sense from spectators that they were waiting for the fall. There was a strong sense that my life was bound to go horribly wrong. I think they wanted me to end up as a crumpled little heap, my feet sticking out from under my guitar – in fact, it often felt as if male music journos thought I had no business even playing a guitar! I think it's to do with being a woman 'plucked from obscurity' (another very odd phrase!). The upshot is that you're often made to feel that you are where you are because you've been granted temporary access. That's quite destabilising and it can make you feel you have to prove yourself, over and over again.

Later in this book, I'll tell you more about the pressures that were on me when I started out in the music business, and how that affected my health and self-perception (the two are so linked, I think). But even though it wasn't plain sailing, I am proud that I was always able to maintain my training and some of my fitness. In many ways, the practice of emotional survival during my childhood had already instilled in me a strong sense of what was dangerous, so I knew that I couldn't go down a route of excess and extreme, and exercise or movement – even a quick jog in the middle of a hectic tour – would be the thing that kept me together.

But I was still far away from being my brightest self. I was using my fitness to keep on the straight and narrow, or to build stamina so that I could work even harder. I wasn't using it for me, and I had not yet been able to work out how to balance my creative process with my rational side. As I mentioned in the introduction to this book, good songwriting comes from a diffucult place – submitting to pain and reliving trauma, not doing squats in the gym or creating smoothie recipes.

I'll get on to the subject of friends later, but for now I just want to say that I love those people who just cut to the chase and are super-honest about you. One day I was working with my friend Nathan, who is my stylist. Our working relationship was fairly new and Nathan seemed somewhat puzzled by the direction of some of my recent looks, which were very much about being incredibly glossy and involved extravagant hair extensions and that kind of thing. 'Can I ask,' he said gently, in a way that I've begun to realise is very Nathan-esque, 'what is your motivation for your look?' *Hmmm*, I thought, *now that is an interesting question*. And just like that, it dawned on me that I was trying to look how I thought the perfect pop princess should look.

I realise this is quite a niche story, but I guarantee you'll have your version of it. We can all get stuck trying to recreate the perfect archetype: wife, mother, singer, performer, surgeon, athlete, you name it. But it pays to be alert to this, because if you're trying to reach perfection as an archeytpe, then as Salvador Dali might have also put it – you're going to fuck it up!

I also think there's a strong link between perfection and fear. That has certainly been my experience. As I was thinking about how to explain this, I began reading *Untamed*, a memoir by the activist, speaker and wonderful writer Glennon Doyle, who majors in the joy and peace we can achieve when we stop trying to meet the expectations of the world around us and start trusting the voice within us (I would highly recommend her books). This sentence from *Untamed* beamed out at me, as if it was backlit: 'What the world needs is more women who have quit fearing themselves and started trusting themselves.' Yasssss, Glennon! This is exactly it!

You simply cannot realise your brightest self if you are dancing to someone else's tune. Same if you are trying to

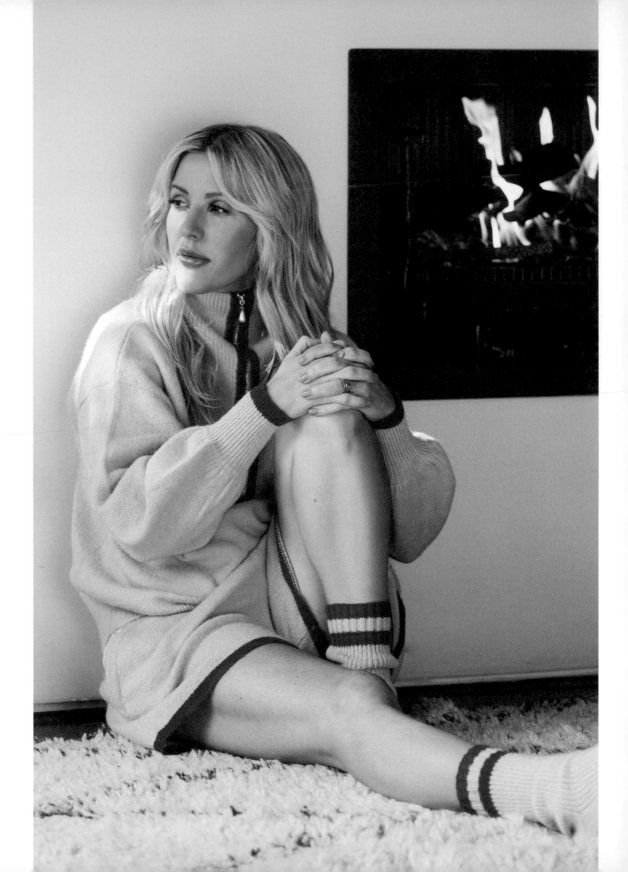

run someone else's race or emulate an influencer's idea of fitness as prescribed by social media. Similarly, fear leads us to associate successful health and fitness with control and deprivation (expressions of fear). What I want us to try doing is to flip that on its head, listen to the voice deep within us and trust ourselves, rather than a lot of external rules and signals created by other people.

That voice, that trust and that confidence adds up to your brightest self.

But we're not going to flick a switch and turn the old you off and the brightest self on – sorry, it doesn't work like that! This is all a work in progress, a spring cleaning to retire old patterns of behaviour and mindsets in favour of moving forwards and – as we go through the chapters – combining physical training with nutrition and the building of emotional resilience. But first I want to set out my ten principles. These are the foundations all of our work will be built on:

1. Swap out perfection for flexibility

I have to admit, I felt quite stupid when I realised the perfection I had dedicated myself to achieving didn't really exist. (I mean, you would, wouldn't you?) But I also felt a tremendous sense of relief. No more 'Oh, I have to be the best singer, the best athlete, the best friend and the best girlfriend of all time blah blah blah.' That realisation came just at the right time because I'm also now a wife and a mum, and I certainly wouldn't have wanted to subject those roles to my perfection quest.

Actually, I don't think you should ever lower your horizons; I strongly believe you should try hard and strive to be the best version of yourself, in all areas of your life – from career to exercise – because it will make you feel good. But swapping out the complete fiction of perfection? Hell, yeah!

Instead you are replacing this with the understanding that you need a flexible, agile approach to life. This is because the flipside of perfection isn't being a chaotic hot mess (sometimes we feel this is where we'll end up if we relinquish control). It is flexibility.

To put that in the context of our work in this book: what you do most of the time is more important than what you do some of the time. Matt Roberts, Pixie Turner and I are not going to hunt you down and read you the Riot Act if you order a takeaway once a week to share with somebody you love. Because that doesn't take away from eating healthy, nourishing meals all the rest of the week. Similarly, skipping a gym session because you've had a bad day at work and didn't sleep well last night doesn't take away from all the other hard work you've put in and the sessions you usually do.

Letting go of perfection is about giving yourself a break. People who strive for perfection – and I've been there, as we've seen – either end up burned out or feeling like they're constantly failing. They do not feel like their brightest selves.

2. What you wear doesn't matter

Closely related to the above abandonment of perfection, this second point mixes a bit of flexibility with courage. Social media has a lot to answer for, especially in the health and fitness space. It can make us feel constrained by a standardised idea of what looks good: this extends from being preoccupied with facial expressions (honestly, I've heard heartbreaking stories of young women refusing to lift heavy weights in case they make funny faces) to obsessing about wearing matching workout sets or limiting workouts to Instagrammable routines with Pecs-McGee trainers who shout motivational phrases while you pretend to be absolutely fine. Let's just bin all of that, shall we?

The truth is, a good workout is ugly and often boring to watch. It's sweaty and, with my skin tones, quite often tomato-faced. Some people are beautiful runners. I am not one of them; somehow I always look like this is my first run. This is probably not enhanced by my greying, fraying gym shorts that have clocked up eight years of service and hundreds of wears. But they're just so damned comfortable! So never let social media (or anything else) lead you to believe you're somehow lacking or less than.

'Resilience: the art of caring for the right things'

MAXIME LAGACE, WRITER

3. Engage your other (mental) core

I wish you understood how resilient you are already! We so often just scrape the surface when it comes to our mental toughness. I know the phrase 'dig deep' is a super-annoying fitness cliché, but honestly it shouldn't just be something you do when you plant trees. There's a moment in every fitness session when we can keep going or we can stop. If you keep going, you will not regret it.

When I talk about 'strength', I am referring to both my physical and my emotional strength – because we need both of these to help us through tough situations. I know from my husband, Caspar, that rowers refer to this point as seeing 'the red mist'. It's where the urge to get to the finish overpowers what you've got left physically. It becomes exclusively about the mind. Caspar describes it like breaking through a barrier where pain is the only thing you feel but because you know you are so close to the finish, you can somehow take it.

I'm not suggesting we have to go this far and go through life seeking out red-mist scenarios! But I'm completely fascinated by the remarkable human mind and the fact that this strength lies dormant in us all. In the introduction to this book I mentioned that Caspar and I use training in really different ways, but here I've definitely learned from him. Whereas I used to say to myself, 'I'm going to avoid that situation because it will make me feel unhappy or take me out of my comfort zone', now I will often say to myself, 'There will always be tough moments so I need to strengthen my mind to navigate calmly through them.'

When you achieve that level of composure in a difficult situation, then it feels like you are really moving forwards. This is summed up perfectly by one of my favourite quotes from the poet and activist Yung Peublo, 'I knew I was on the right path when I started feeling peace in situations I would normally feel tension'.

But while inner strength and resilience is important, acknowledging our weaknesses and vulnerability is also fundamental. So I also think it's important to acknowledge that it's completely OK to feel uncomfortable in situations when society or peers seem to think you should breeze through. I've had to be around big crowds most of my adult life, and yet sometimes I get so nervous I'm seriously afraid I'm going to throw up. (A really good way to handle these moments is to tell someone in the same position and nine times out of ten they will confess to feeling exactly the same. There's nothing like an ally when you're scared out of your wits!)

Following a tricky situation where you felt very uncomfortable, take time to reflect without tearing yourself apart about it. What is of use is understanding why you felt so nervous in that room of people, or why you might have started an argument. Throughout this book we'll use those types of reflections because they are of great value in navigating your future.

4. Be as kind to yourself as you are to your best friend

In the past, the way I sometimes spoke to myself was frankly unacceptable. So I asked myself why would I let myself get away with negative, self-talk – if I had a friend who did that, I would give them their friendship P45? (By the way, my real friends are absolutely legends and I'll talk about the importance of having them in my life in a little more detail later on.)

But there's a huge difference between being intensely hard on ourselves and gently taking the piss out of ourselves. The latter has been a life saver for me. I'm forever finding parallels with me in pop-star scenarios and scenes from *Extras* or *Alan Partridge*. I have laughed at myself (often by myself) in pretty much every country on Earth, often on live TV, and I'm glad I did because without that stress release I would have most likely fallen apart.

But overall try and be as kind to yourself as you are to your best friend. Acknowledge your achievements, no matter how small. And remember it's all about progression, not perfection.

Try this exercise: ask yourself, what do I like about myself? What am I good at? How would my best friends describe me? (It's OK: you can do this in the privacy of your own room rather than out loud on the bus.) I saw a therapist* recently, who did this exercise with me. She asked me questions like 'Would you say you were kind?' and 'Would your friends describe you as kind?' Initially I did that typical British thing of feeling embarrassed and trying to make a joke about being a terrible person, but then I surprised myself by really thinking about

* By the way, if it's very British to love self-deprecating comedy like *Alan Partridge*, but it is decidedly un-British to talk about accessing professional psychotherapy. I consider myself really lucky to have the means to access a professional therapist periodically. In fact, I think is one of the best investments I've made in my wellbeing. If you feel this route is for you, be sure to find a therapist who is accredited.

the therapist's questions and answering them honestly. I was taken aback by what a difference it made to how I was feeling. I thought, *I really do care about my friends, and I really do think I'm good at these things*. I would almost describe it as revelatory!

5. Remember, you are the gatekeeper

I want you to imagine a roped-off VIP area in an old-fashioned club. (Over lockdown, I have genuinely caught myself longing to be in a smelly, sticky club.) The rope is one of those thick red ones and there's a bouncer on a power trip who decides who is let into this area by looking them up and down and unhooking the rope to let them in. The burly bouncer? That's you! But this space is both your mind and your diary. Who you let in defines how you're going to spend your day. If you fill this space with horrible brawling or boring people, you're going to have a shit day. So choose wisely!

As you're the gatekeeper for your mind, you can choose what you let in. Just as food is there to nourish the body (see below), this is the stuff that fuels your mind. Whether it's social media, sugar, excessive working, too much exercise – you are under no obligation to let this stuff in. Indeed, ultimately, as you know these are bad for you, it's completely logical that you would choose to limit them.

While I'm not averse to the odd evening watching the *Real Housewives* format from any number of geographical locations, I do believe we also need access to high-quality, intelligent opinion and trusted impartial news organisations. I like to hear from educators and people who empower me and help me prioritise the things that are super-important to me. That's the reason I don't fill up my days watching online clips of angry people full of hate and it's the reason I am trying to limit scrolling on social media. My inner bouncer says *Not on the list, love*.

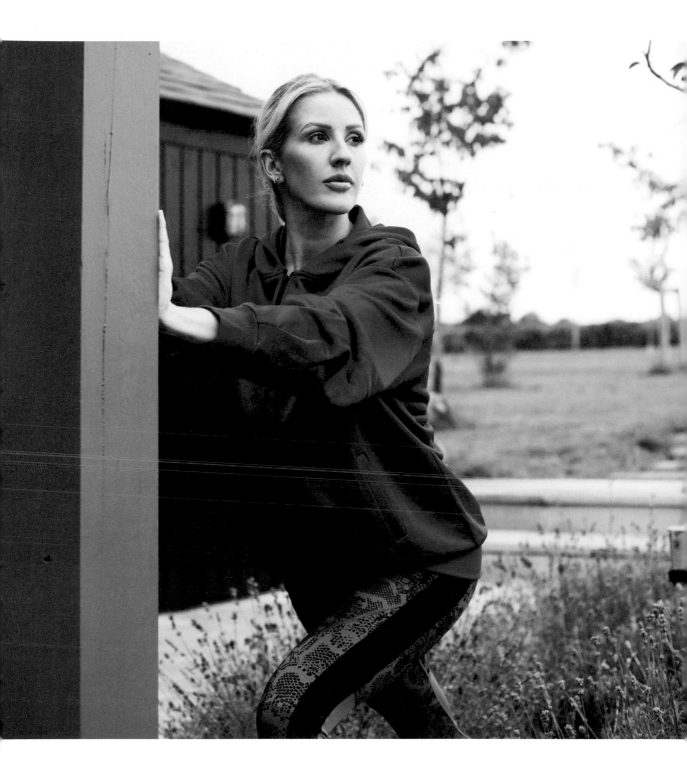

'There are times when your only available tools are your mind and your breath'

CATHERINE CARRIGAN, MEDICAL INTUITIVE HEALER AND AUTHOR

6. Get serious about breathing

A surprising amount of my songs feature lyrics about breathing (the same is true of other artists' songs, too). I think I might be a bit obsessed, but then I wonder why more of us aren't into breathing beyond just staying alive?! Inhaling deeply and taking that breath right down to oxygenate the whole body is a secret superpower that can boost your training capacity. Yet again, breathing well is an example of something we turn to in times of crisis – demonstrations by doctors of breathing techniques went viral in the early days of Covid-19 – but rarely get talked about in everyday life.

I think this is an oversight. Every time someone mentions breathing, I find myself taking a really deep breath. Not just an instinctive shallow breath where we only half-fill our upper chest, but a full breath that feels like it has passed through every cell in the body. It seems way too easy, but it really is the most simple but effective way of bringing ourselves back into the moment, when we're caught moping in the past or future.

When I had my first panic attack (which I'll talk more about in the next chapter), I took myself to hospital, convinced I was having a heart attack and expecting to be hooked up to machines. Instead, I was simply given a paper bag and told to 'breathe, breathe'.

Whenever I feel stressed, I think about this moment. It's such a clear reminder of the power of our breath and how learning to control it can help our nervous system and calm our senses. In Chapter 6, 'Find Your Strength' barre supremo Catie Miller is going to talk you through a really powerful breathing exercise.

I'd love you to remember that breathing can be used for much more than just filling our lungs to survive. Our breath is intrinsically linked to our physical and mental wellbeing and learning how to breathe properly can transform your health. Never forget that you have it at your disposal, whenever you might need it.

7. Food is your fuel

We'll talk about food a lot in this book. We'll look at our relationship with it, my relationship with it and how this often needs fixing (especially in Chapter 4, 'Nourish Your Body'). But I want to make some key points now, as these are central to the way I think about health and fitness overall.

Food gives us energy, sustenance and the strength to move our bodies and get through the day. We need to eat, and we need to eat well. I don't think deprivation is ever the answer, especially when it comes to food. Food is there to make us better and stronger, happier and healthier. It nourishes your body and it fuels your muscles. But that only works if you eat the right things.

I believe it's so important to understand what we're putting into our bodies and the effect this has on our physical and mental wellbeing. As much pleasure as a chocolate bar (or a takeaway) brings (and I've felt that that x1000 during pregnancy), it doesn't last as long as the feeling you get when you eat healthy, nourishing food. Be mindful of foods that offer fast but temporary gratification and educate yourself on the benefits of a good diet. The more you learn about the powerful nutritional and emotional benefits of food, the more you'll want to eat well – and enjoy the process of preparing food, too.

Food is also a complete joy. It binds us to people and can bring comfort in a very healthy way. I'm imagining a Sunday roast, for example. It's delicious, but also heartwarming and good for the soul. It's also the one time other than Christmas Day when I actually like to be uncomfortably full. A dinner party with wine similarly offers a moment of escape with friends. (How much did we miss that during the long lockdowns of the global pandemic?) In almost every culture, food forms a central part of celebration; that means for billions of humans food is at the heart of their most cherished memories on earth.

But healthy food can also be joyful! And I think that fact is often ignored. The other day, I made an acai bowl for breakfast and it brought me an embarrassing amount of pleasure – I had to text at least five people to let them know – sorry, guys. I had it with goji berries (which are sweet and madly good for you), hemp protein, cacao nibs (which give you a burst of energy), blueberries, raspberries and chia seeds. I threw it all in the bowl; it was so simple to make, and not only did it taste like heaven but it overachieved on 'five a day' health advice and then some! (Yep, I get competitive about my fruit and veg goals!) And yet, I often have to keep this nutritional superiority quiet to avoid offending those who subsist on sugar and make 'rabbit food' comments when I mention vegan ingredients. I also resent it when people almost shame others for taking pride in their love for healthy food. If you're having junk food – good for you! But don't mock someone for legitimately enjoying something that is a bit healthier!

Well, the good news is there's no keeping quiet in this book. All the recipes in Chapter 8, 'How I Eat: The Recipes' are super-healthy and nutritious, but – and this bit was really important for me when I was writing this book – also delicious and joyful, and great to share with friends and people you love.

8. Ditch the comparisons

Were I ever to hold significant office with law-making capability (unlikely, I know), first off I'd ban perfectionism (see above), and next I'd ban 'comparisons'. Every journey is individual, so never compare yours to someone else's. It is simply not useful.

Nor – when we come to health and fitness – is it credible. We've all been brought up differently, with our own childhood and influences along the way. We all have different genetic make-ups, we store fat differently, we have different hormone levels, different body shapes, different likes and dislikes, different fitness levels, different pain thresholds and different motivations. That is why life is unique for all of us. So, for example, mindlessly eating the same food as someone else you admire the look of really doesn't work. You need to listen to and understand your own body (a subject we'll move on to soon).

At this point I'm going to return to the subject of social media. I find a lot of people's comparison obsession takes place on Instagram these days and there are reasons to be really careful of this. Social-media platforms such as Instagram can distort our reality, according to psychology researchers such as Danielle Wagstaff from the Federation University in Australia. I came across a fascinating article where Danielle describes the way in which our brain compares the images of influencers that we follow to create a schema (a cognitive representation of your sense of self and of other people). 'Back in the day your social circle was formed of friends and family,' she explained in the piece. 'Now you have access to all of these influencers. That means our perceived social circle is enormous. It would be too exhausting to make a judgement every time you saw a new image of someone from this circle, so cognitively your mind automatically creates an average.' But the problem with this average, according to Danielle is that all the images you're exposed to on social media are highly curated and edited – even no-filter, no-make-up shots are selected – meaning that the 'average' that your brain creates is not a true representation of someone's lifestyle, attractiveness or income. 'If you're constantly being presented with false information or information that is biased, then your schema is biased. It doesn't represent the real world,' she concludes.

9. The destination is not the point

I used to fixate on making songs that would chart high, blagging the best outfits I could, and always trying to be on top, because anything less wasn't good enough. But then came the dawning realisation that this strategy completely missed the point. In fact, it meant I was bypassing the thing that gave me joy in the first place – the creativity, the process and the very thing my craft is based on: noticing what is going on around me, listening to people and taking things in. I was able to recalibrate and reprioritise my creativity. The more I focused on enjoying every moment – even the boring moments! – the more the good stuff started to come naturally.

This is my way of emphasising that rather than obsessing about an end goal, you need to make the journey, this journey, part of your process and enjoy it as part of your achievement.

It's great to run a 5 or a 10k, or maybe lose the weight you weren't happy about, but I would advise that you don't worry too much about achieving an end goal. In fact, my hope is that we forget big health goals, and start thinking about good health as a sustainable, long-term way of living. I really believe there is so much satisfaction and peace of mind when you know you made extra effort to become a stronger version of yourself.

10. Hold yourself accountable

This might sound a bit tough, and a bit like something a teacher might have said to you at school, but it is truly liberating to acknowledge that you are accountable for your own health and wellbeing. At the risk of sounding a bit weird, I almost think of it like I've signed a contract with myself. (I'm not talking about making it a big deal like the Magna Carta, with trumpets and a formal declaration at Runnymede.) But even a tacit acknowledgement to yourself that you are on the case here will work. What are you committing to? Well, just to knowing that there is no magical force at work here; this is not luck, but consistent commitment and hard work, will really help you to turn all of this self-knowledge and hard work into consistent progress.

And the truth is that from time to time you'll lose your mojo and motivation; we all do. You'll eat a doughnut instead of going for a run. Good. A) thank you for keeping me company in the being-very-human-stakes, and b) you may well have needed it. But because you're in a serious relationship with your fitness, and you've made this contract, you will always have that link back. You will correct your course, pick up your routine and re-commit. Because that's what you do!

I really find this helpful because for me it's about approaching everything in a connected, sustainable and balanced way – these are ways of being and living that you will stick with for the long term, and it should feel great to know and understand that.

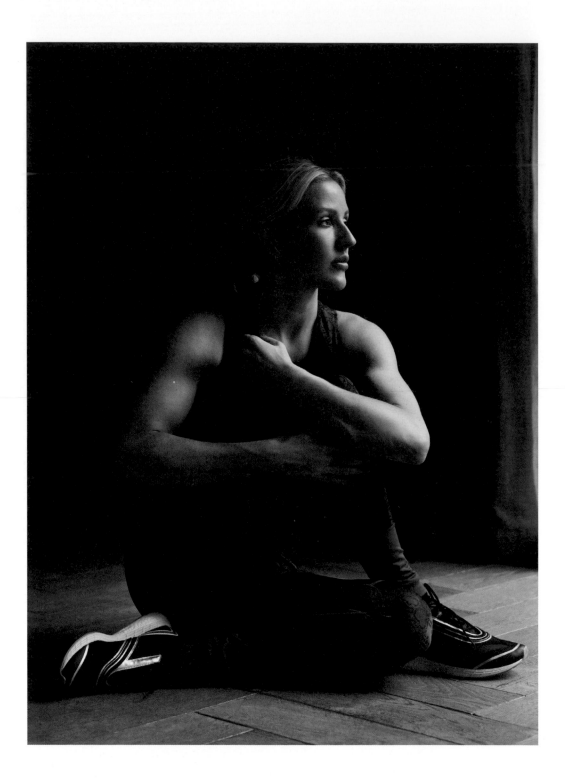

2 LISTEN TO YOUR BODY

'If you listen to your body when it whispers,
you won't have to hear it scream'

ANON

Are you at war with your body? It's a weird question, but it's one that's worth asking because many of us are. Instead of listening attentively – and our bodies are really well placed to know what's going on – we often ignore what our bodies are trying to tell us. Then to add insult to injury, we actively find ways of sabotaging them. This can be subtle or overt. But we come up with myriad ways to carry this out. Common ambushes include running ourselves into the ground by overworking; failing to move for hours on end from sedentary environments where we're hunched over laptops; flooding our bodies with anxiety and stress (and therefore adrenaline and cortisol) at completely random times; failing to prioritise sleep; and then trying to make everything OK by shovelling in rubbish food (and we have the audacity to call this 'comfort food'). Oh dear.

I'm guilty of doing all of this. There were countless times I shushed that little voice inside my head – and my gut – that was desperately trying to warn me I was exercising too much, taking on too much at work, or becoming anxious and stressed. In fact, I allowed myself to become drained to the point I was having panic attacks (in this chapter I describe how and why I think this came about). If my body was a hotel at that time, it would have had one of the crappiest Trip Advisor ratings ever. 'Appalling management. I will never stay here again. PS: Rubbish wifi signal in rooms.'

Yet on the surface things would have looked perfectly fine. Remember, I was keeping up my training and fitness (that self-preservation that got me through the tough times kicked in) and I was probably quite buff – even if I didn't think so at the time. This serves to reinforce that critical point: muscles and fitness are not enough by themselves. In order to achieve a really useful level of health and wellbeing, you absolutely have to work with your body, not in opposition to it.

That means listening to it. I can't say that too many times. Because rather than listening carefully to our bodies we have a tendency to suppress warning signs. We often wait until there's a fully fledged crisis before we act. So in this chapter we're going to explore doing the opposite – acting now, listening really intensely – and we're even going to try and get some data on what your body is telling you. This is something I'm really interested in because it's much easier to change what you've measured and written down. And once you have those data they can form a goldmine. You know when you're progressing and you can also get advanced warning when things are going awry. Our bodies, in effect, provide our own evidence base. But only, of course, if we listen to them.

I appreciate that's a lot of skills if you're learning from scratch, but I promise you it's one of the most transformative set of skills I have learned.

OVERWORKING

I'm just going to take this opportunity to elaborate a little bit on the subject of overworking. Because I think taking too much on is probably one of the most common forms of self-sabotage and one of the most common forms of tuning out when your body is telling you not to push. It is also super-connected to all the things we discussed in Chapter 1. But just as you can surrender the quest for perfection without turning into a chaotic heap, you will not turn into a human sloth when you start implementing boundaries, distinguishing between work hours and living time (something we've all allowed to blur during lockdowns) and being realistic about what you can take on. The solution to overworking is not underworking. It's not like you can say to your line manager, 'Actually, you know what, I'm going to relax today.' I work for myself on paper, but in reality I serve an audience. They are everything to me, so I'm not going to suddenly appear on stage shouting 'Good evening, Wembley!

I'm going to put in 40 per cent effort tonight because I want to save my energy for something I'm doing later in the week.' (Actually even writing that makes me feel really weird.) I love playing to my audience, and I love playing to other people's audiences – sometimes you have to get a crowd on your side and I will throw every last drop of energy at it. Lockdown sucked for everyone, but as a performer, oh my goodness, I cannot tell you how much I missed performing! Coming back, I'm not planning to put in any 'meh' performances, I can tell you. But the point is, I won't need to. When you learn to listen to your body, you regulate yourself, you make really good decisions about what to prioritise and what to take on, stop being available to everyone all the time and that leaves you free to kill those big moments and excel at your real job.

How I made it – and how it nearly broke me

At the age of nineteen I was spotted by a music manager called Jamie Lillywhite and I decided to leave university early to see if I could make a career out of my music. I found a little room to rent in a house in Hammersmith and managed to borrow a small amount of money that I'd rather optimistically thought would fund my new life. My priorities were food, sleep, my guitar, a few good books and membership of a cheap gym down the road.

Oh, it was hard, especially the isolation. This was probably the most solitary time of my life. I'd left the few friends I did have at university behind and decided to try London alone. There was no safety net. No Plan B. Without much money, I was constantly waiting for record labels to get back to me. I spent a lot of time running and strength training in the gym. It's so weird to think that I was completely oblivious to the fact that just over a year later everything, *and I mean everything*, would change.

As 2009 came to an end, I signed to the record label Polydor. Here was a label that really believed in me. I released a few songs. A year later, at the age of twenty-four, that clutch of songs had grown into my debut album, *Lights*. It won me my first Brit Award and took me to number one in the UK album charts. It was like being strapped to a space shuttle. I found myself performing live on TV, going to awards ceremonies and sometimes flying to three countries in a day. Let's just say that again: *three countries in a day*. It was a total whirlwind. Yes, it was a dream come true because I was so passionate about singing and writing songs, and had been from childhood. But you have to accept that brilliant things can also be detrimental. It was also why, by my mid-twenties, I ended up suffering from debilitating panic attacks.

My panic attacks began to build slowly. I remember experiencing one on an early photoshoot. Of course, I couldn't name it as a panic attack because it was new to me. I just knew that I felt quite strange. I had a feeling of unease building up inside my body. It happened again shortly afterwards when I was about to take part in a live TV show. I did the show. I acted my way through it, as if me going on live TV while having an enormous yet secret panic attack was the most normal thing in the world. I was acting the part of the pop star, but inside none of it felt real or deserved. To this day I have never watched that show back. I'm scared I will spot the terror in my eyes.

In fact, my twenties felt like a combination of complete euphoria and utter terror. My main thoughts seemed to run like this: *This isn't real. Is this real? I don't deserve this! This a complete fluke. Did they get the wrong person?* Etc., etc. On a near-continuous loop, these thoughts are exhausting.

I now know this relentless dialogue to be one of the chief signs of Impostor Syndrome. This is a syndrome described by psychologists Pauline Rose Clance and Suzanne Imes nearly half a century ago. There's some debate as to whether it should be classified as a mental-health disorder (to date it hasn't been) and of course some debate whether it is actually real. All I can say is, it felt pretty real to me. According to Clance and Imes's original research your early family dynamics play a big part in determining whether you suffer from Impostor Syndrome. They also said that you were more likely to experience it if you were a woman, and particularly if you were a Black or Asian woman. This is because societal sex-roles and racial stereotyping also play a role. Recent research, however, says that men are just as likely to suffer from Impostor Syndrome in work-related environments. I was really interested when I quizzed Caspar, my husband, who seems unshakeably confident, that he had also experienced it. I suppose we can console ourselves with the knowledge that even Einstein was a sufferer. He once proclaimed that 'the exaggerated esteem in which my lifework is held makes me very ill at ease. I feel compelled to think of myself as an involuntary swindler.'

Putting a name to anguish and unease, and understanding that you're not the only one, is a really helpful way to navigate through these attacks. I wish I had thought to talk to people about how I was feeling at the time. I also wish I had spent more time acknowledging that what was happening to me and around me was totally bizarre. But I didn't because I always felt it was the wrong time to bring that up. And besides, life was moving at a frenetic pace and I felt I had to say yes to everything all of the time.

One day, a close friend from back home in Hereford called to say her dad had passed away. As a kid, this family had provided me with lots of support and refuge from home, when I wasn't getting on well there. I was devastated for my friend, and I wanted to support her, so I told my team I was taking my first days off to go to the funeral of my friend's dad. Sitting on the train, I also realised: this was the first time I had sat still in two years.

In that moment of quiet, on a trundling train, on my own, with nobody around to tell me what to do, the enormity of everything struck me. Panic began to rise up from the pit of my stomach to the back of my throat and then, just at that point, the train jolted and broke down – a depressingly perfect symbol of how I felt. When the rail-replacement service buses failed to turn up, I ended up in a taxi with a few of the other passengers. I felt hot and cold. My heart was racing. I heard a small voice say 'Err, excuse me, I think I'm having a heart attack.' I realised the small voice was mine. A very sweet woman instructed the taxi to head for the nearest hospital. In A&E a doctor diagnosed a bad panic attack.

I'd love to say we solved the issue then and there, but instead of listening to my body and coming up with a way of processing all that was happening, I normalised the attacks. They became kind of routine. Some days it was just a quiet, sickly feeling in my heart that sent waves of cold panic through my body, often accompanied by feelings of dread. Other times an attack could spiral into a full and frightening physical manifestation. If anybody reading this is unlucky enough to have suffered panic attacks, then you will know how utterly terrifying they are.

For reasons of shame and confusion (I had chosen this career so I felt I should carry on with it), it took me a long time to seek help. Eventually I found Cognitive Behavioural Therapy (CBT). This is defined by the NHS as 'a talking therapy that can help you manage your problems by changing the way you think and behave'.* For me, it was life changing. I can't tell you how much it helped to speak to someone who was totally impartial. My therapist taught me to listen to my inner voice and to validate my own feelings, rather than looking for external

---

* It is a source of real concern for me that CBT isn't easier to access on the NHS and that many of those who need it have to wait for so long to access a therapist. But there are free-to-call services if you are in crisis, or close to someone who is, so please access help. I have listed some at the end of this book.

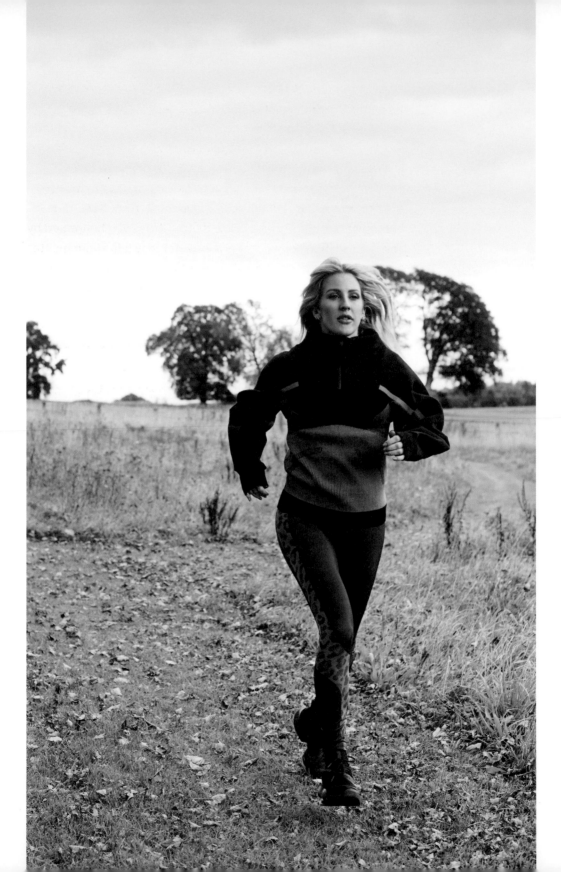

validation or trying to supress them. One of the things I really remember is that crying suddenly seemed like a beautiful release, rather than a sign of weakness.

I believe everyone should have access to good mental health professionals who can help them navigate the huge pressures that life brings today. It breaks my heart that not everyone is able to access the services that helped me so much and find a therapist who they really click with. I am, however, heartened by the huge shift in the way that we now actually talk about mental health because it used to be a taboo. I can't say this strongly enough: we all have the right to feel the way we do, whoever we are and whatever we have.

I don't think I would have had the confidence to share these thoughts with you a few years ago. There was a sense that if you were a celebrity, any troubles you had were of your own making (similar to the warped logic that caused my panic attacks) and that if you said anything people would respond by making jokes about tiny violins, etc.

What I learned through working with a therapist is that every feeling counts. It's easy to look at a famous person, or somebody who has a seemingly perfect life with a big house, beautiful healthy children or a good job, and think *What have you got to be sad about?* (And this is pretty similar to leaning out of your van and saying 'Cheer up, love, it might never happen'.) But as anybody who has suffered from depression or anxiety will know, those things don't cushion you. What finally helped me was being able to process my thoughts and to talk freely about how I felt.

MY TOP THREE TIPS

- Remember that your feelings matter. It doesn't matter what you have – money, fame, family, a new baby, a great job. If you feel sad, those feelings are real and valid, so listen to them.

- Listen to your body when it's telling you to slow down. We're human, we're not robots and we will burn out if we don't listen to that voice telling us to slow down occasionally.

- Seek help if you need it. There is no shame in seeing a therapist if you feel your problems are spiralling and becoming too much for you to process. Friends and family are great sounding boards, but I like the fact that a therapist is impartial and separate from everything else going on in my life.

Is there such a thing as too much exercise?

'Please, please, please can I have more time for running?' This was the question I asked my manager on an almost hourly basis. As I began to recover from my panic attacks, fitness became my sanctuary. My manager carved out thirty minutes during the working day when I could exercise. This might sound a little stingy, but given our schedule – recording, interviews, live TV, travelling – it was heroic of him to give me this. This was my golden half hour. Working in such a busy, full-on and unpredictable industry, it was the one time where I could switch off with no one around. (Another thing about training is that you can plug in your headphones and it's not rude!)

Unfortunately, it wasn't long before exercise became my prison. It seemed all I could think about was when my next workout was going to be. I didn't realise it at the time, but I was clearly using exercise as a crutch. I couldn't control many things around me, but I could control how much I exercised.

I went back to my manager, demanding more 'down-time' – which was code in my head for pushing myself to the limit on a treadmill. This workout time became quite the bone of contention between us, with me constantly demanding more time from the schedule. I think the poor guy was a bit bemused by it all.

I'd land in a country, get to the hotel at 11 p.m. and I'd be on the treadmill by midnight. If I had an early evening work meeting with a couple of drinks, I'd jump on when I got back to the hotel. OK, I wasn't raging drunk, but it wasn't exactly ideal.

Exercising too much led me to start eating poorly as well. Rather than seeing food as fuel and making wise decisions, I'd eat rubbish and think I could just burn off the calories (rather than thinking how I was going to use them). I didn't see the value of food or even consider how my eating could benefit my training or help me to train better. In my case it wasn't about weight and being super-thin (as I know this kind of pattern of behaviour often can be); it was about distracting myself from how I felt.

I am fully aware this is not the most rock and roll account of wanton destruction. I wasn't mainlining drugs and chucking white goods out of hotel windows, or eating the heads off pigeons or anything. Sorry if that's a bit disappointing – but to be fair you have bought a book titled *Fitter. Calmer. Stronger.* so I'm not sure what you were expecting. Perhaps that's why my colleagues (many of whom are dear friends) didn't spot that I wasn't just super-fit but running myself into the ground. Many had been in the music business for a while and were probably looking out for different signs of worrying behaviour than a singer who seems to like a bit of running.

But it's all relative, isn't it? Addiction to anything sneaks up on you, sends false signals and starts to unravel you. Being on a treadmill at midnight, pounding away and pouring with sweat when you're exhausted isn't fun and it's not healthy.

Besides, it was exhausting. Not necessarily the exercise, where at least for the first part of this period I was excelling. I was crazy strong. I could lift heavier weights than any other woman I knew. And my endurance was off the chart. I could outrun and out-lift everyone around me. I was always the last one standing in a HIIT session. No, it was more the stress of constantly competing with myself to be fitter that was really exhausting. I would beat myself up if I underperformed in the gym, the same way I would if I felt I hadn't had a good performance on stage, or if my voice was off. I now realise I was burning out.

As has happened at other points in my life, I suddenly woke up to what was going on. In this way I was able to avert a total crisis. There was no dramatic realisation or moment it all became clear to me, just a sense that from loving my training and finding a sanctuary, I was beginning to actively dislike it. But to give up on the very thing that had sustained me for so long would have been a real tragedy for me. Besides, it was obvious from looking around that it was possible to have a healthy relationship with diet and fitness, and in fact these things could underpin a happy and productive life. As I began to slow down, even occasionally doing nothing (a state which I now cherish), I became determined that I would find a way of balancing all of this so that healthy living was truly healthy and where my physical and mental health could support my life without completely defining it.

WHAT DOES AN UNHEALTHY RELATIONSHIP WITH EXERCISE LOOK LIKE?

- Do you feel stressed or guilty if you can't make it to the gym or go for a run?
- Do you vow to eat less because you've had to miss a workout? Or work out for longer or harder to 'make up' for food you've eaten?
- Do you cancel plans to see friends or family so you can work out?
- Do you make sure you never miss a workout, even if you're tired, unwell, hungover or injured?
- Do you exercise at unsociable times (for example, very late at night) in order to make sure you fit it in?

If you have answered yes to any of the above questions, then speak to your GP.

Of course, change on this level, with deeply ingrained patterns of behaviours, is easier said than done. These are the things I did to change course:

- Slowed down to the extent that I sometimes 'did nothing', which also included reading a book (which is of course 'doing something', but you get my point!).
- If I was feeling stressed, I would swap a run for a gentle yoga session.
- If I felt overwhelmed, I would go for a gentle jog in a park, focusing on breathing and keeping my pace slow.
- Only when I felt well rested, had eaten properly and felt like I had the necessary reserves of energy would I allow myself to go all out with a fast run or HIIT session.

Do you remember in the last chapter, I rounded off my ten core princples with 'Hold Yourself Accountable'? In my experience, it was only when I finally became able to listen that I was able to take accountability. As Jon Kabat-Zinn, a US academic who specialises in stress reduction and mindfulness puts it, 'Nobody can listen to your body for you. To grow and heal you have to take responsibility for listening to it yourself.'

So while I had broken the pattern that had led me to over-exercise with this strategy, there was still a lot more work to do in order to avoid falling back into old habits, or even abandoning fitness altogether. I wanted to reset from a much healthier place. I started reading about the subject much more and watching online videos from incredible experts. I wasn't just learning new ways of exercising, I was listening to TED talks on the connection between psychology and physiology and the emerging world of biohacking. I found it so inspiring.

All of these professionals were, in a sense, talking about listening to your body rather than imposing some random rules on it. I decided to follow their advice. This entailed quietly ditching strange vows that I had made to myself. One of these was that I didn't need a trainer. For years, despite being increasingly in the public eye and making friends with lots of people in my industry who recommended trainers (because they knew I loved sport and fitness), I was adamant I could do it alone. Looking back, that's kind of weird. Perhaps I just didn't want a professional to analyse what I was doing too closely because they'd know I was over-exercising.

After I burned out through over-exercising, I had to reverse this decision. I had to admit that I needed someone to help me with my approach to training. I had started coming back slowly, but honestly I found it a bit frustrating. I knew that I'd got into an unhealthy place with exercise and I didn't want to go back there, but God, I missed what I thought were spectacular results (I still didn't realise I'd be able to get better results from a healthy approach). On some level, I thought if

I had a trainer, I would get back to my fittest-person-on-the-planet thing.

This wasn't the most noble reason admittedly, but I'll let that one go! The fact is, I met Matt Roberts, who has become a big part of my life and who I will talk about more in Chapter 7 when he introduces a special set of workouts for us.

As soon as I began training with Matt, things began to click into place. It was pretty evident that he wasn't there just to let me obsess about hollow goals. What struck me immediately was the way he was so flexible in his approach. He plans my workouts based on my energy, my mood and what I'm doing for the rest of that day. If I'm not listening to my body properly, then he is! My schedule is still all over the place – I've come to realise it's a hazard of the job. Seeing Matt in the gym is almost an escape for me. But a full and busy life should be unpredictable and varied. Isn't that the point?!

What has changed is that surfing the ups and downs of life has become key to how I approach training. It's connected, rather than a siloed bit of the day. When we feel energised, the HIIT class is manageable. At other times our jobs can get in the way of self-care. Sometimes we're short of sleep and low on energy. If we're travelling or on the go, it can be impossible to maintain a healthy diet. There are good days and bad days and times when mentally we don't feel motivated. And sometimes, we might just be too hungover for that 2k run. There's no one-size-fits-all with exercise. Some days you need to go gently and some days you need to skip it altogether and rest.

I've realised that doing a HIIT or heavy weights session just isn't compatible with a bad night's sleep, a tough week at work or several days on the road eating junk. The point is that I am now taking the cues as to how I train direct from how my body feels and what I need. That is the difference.

Making it really personal

We've established that listening to your body means getting to know your body better and that there are huge advantages to that; you'll be able to read the signals that your body is sending you about your health more fluently and to make better decisions about your wellness. But what if we could super-charge this and *really* get to know what's going on from our hormone levels through to our sleep patterns? Well, increasingly we can as 'wellness' becomes personalised.

This is where I get really excited about what lies ahead – I don't just mean in this book (although that too, obviously) but in our lifetimes. Essentially we're on the cusp of a new era of health, one where tracking our data about how our body is working in real time means that we can make personalised interventions on diet, on training, sleep and even stress levels. And that's just the beginning. This isn't just *listening* to your body, it's *knowing* your body.

We'll hold off the formal introduction to Dr Tamsin Lewis until Chapter 5, where she gives us some great insight into positive mindset. But for now I'll just tell you that Dr Tam (as I like to call her) is a psychologist and neuroscientist who also happens to compete as a top-level triathlete (I know, she's unbelievable). She's also passionate about this new frontier of health. She's helped me to begin to incorporate elements of STEM TECH ('STEM' being the acronym for science, tech, engineering and maths) into my health story.

Because I've found it so empowering, I'm writing about it here. That's despite the fact that you might have got the idea these breakthroughs are out of reach or for fancy athletes or the type of guys who hover-board to meetings in Silicon Valley. But I believe many of us can benefit. At its most simple level, this might involve tracking our heart rate during a workout and using the data to respond in a smart and focused way.

In a sense you can make this as simple or as complicated as you like! You might have heard of biohacking. It's used broadly to describe all sorts of do-it-yourself biology interventions that promise to maximise your ability to realise all sorts of goals, from losing weight to having a better memory. But I don't recommend that you run off in pursuit of those goals. What I want us to think about is how we can implement some ideas from biohacking (hacking the hack, if you like) to help us with our mission here: a sustainable and balanced approach to your health and fitness that makes you feel great.

You may be wearing a fitness tracker already. We'll talk about 'wearables' later on, too. My friends profess to either love them or loathe them, but I do think as a society we are increasingly comfortable using them to track a run, monitor sleep patterns or even stress levels. (By the way, I do think it's important not to become too devoted to your data. Honestly, nobody wants to discuss your sleep patterns at a dinner party – not even myself or Dr Tam!)

As you know, my ambition is that you use this book for the long term. So you might scoff at a wearable now, but in the very near future you could be sporting a ring that is actually getting under your skin and reading your body's unique response to different foods in real time. Also, think about how useful that is on a practical level. No more aimlessly pushing your trolley around the supermarket aisles hoping for divine nutritional inspiration. Instead, you'll be directed by your tracker to the energy sources that are going to best cater for your body's fuelling needs at that moment. Wow!

Admittedly right now you need deep pockets for some of this tech (I'm hoping that will improve too as it mainstreams), but here's a short guide to the biohacks that Dr Tam and I have found helpful, and reasonably accessible so far:

TESTING

If you're looking for the full works that can include tests for your blood, your immune system and even your oxygen-carrying capacity, this will likely set you back hundreds of pounds. But Dr Tam suggests using a specific test to give a snapshot of a particular problem – if not available through your doctor, a specific lab test costs around £150. Dr Tam suggests the tests worth asking your doctor for are: Iron; B12; thyroid; fasting blood sugar; and morning cortisol.

After I began suffering from fatigue after working out, Dr Tam suggested I get a test to give me a snapshot of my iron levels. They revealed I had low iron levels, which in turn revealed that I was pregnant – pretty big news! (I discovered that fatigue and low iron levels are common but sneaky symptoms of pregnancy.) This test meant that aside from discovering that my world was about to be turned upside down by becoming a mum, I could also correct my iron levels. One treatment boosted my iron to optimum levels for the next twelve months.

Dr Tam also pointed me towards using a glucose monitor. I described the fancy ring version above, but there are a few different types on the market, ranging from around £50 to £160. The Freestyle Libre sensor has a good reputation. These were invented for people who suffer from diabetes, allowing them to flash-monitor glucose levels alongside the more traditional method of pricking your finger and testing the blood (they test slightly different things). Depending on your health authority, if you have a diagnosis of diabetes or insulin resistance, you may be able to get a sensor on the NHS.

I don't have a health diagnosis around my glucose levels, but I am aware that they bounce around all over the place. I found wearing a sensor – you pop it on the back of your arm or on your tummy – to be revelatory, when I looked back at the data (collected via an app). When we listen to our bodies closely, we are aware of course that our mood often changes when our blood glucose levels fluctuate. But against the hullaballoo of everyday life it's pretty hard to get precise about when this is happening and what's causing it. Unless of course you've just downed a bag of sweets, in which case you probably don't need to bother Sherlock Holmes.

One of the great things that using a glucose tracker taught me is that some foods we think are cast-iron-clad health wins are actually a total disaster. How many times, for instance, have you been told that porridge is the most healthy way you can start your day? I blame Goldilocks. But as Dr Tam explained to me, for some people it's a disaster, as they convert porridge to sugar super-fast. Well, who knew? And who would know unless they tracked their response? This doesn't mean you have to give up porridge (or anything else) that causes a spike, but adjust to even things out – when it comes to porridge, you might add nuts or coconut cream to balance.

My own trip-hazard, in terms of food, turned out to be smoothies – the thing I assumed was earning me my perfect-princess nutrition badge. Yes, while I thought I was being super-healthy by loading my smoothie with bananas and dates, the insulin tracker provided incontrovertible evidence that they were sending my levels off the charts. We looked at the data, and we modified. I still love a smoothie (there's just something so great about whizzing all of those ingredients up) but now I am more balanced about what goes in. I include some protein in the form of nuts, especially almonds, and that gives me a delicious smoothie without the insulin spike. The goal for me is to avoid a glucose crash and achieve sustained blood glucose levels.

Interventions do not have to be huge or costly or even particularly high tech. Dr Tam is a fan of the sauna blanket, which she says calms your body and mind while detoxifying you (increasingly we're exposed to a cocktail of toxins on a minute-by-minute basis, especially if you live in a city). While some of the infra-red models weigh in at hundreds of pounds, you can get basic models for under £100. Or you can take a hot bath with Epsom salts, which has a similar effect.

The geeky side of my nature means I would love to go on about this stuff all day. Indeed, working with Dr Tam I have embraced different areas of biohacking and started to feel completely different. But to go deep, I think it pays to work with an expert because there is so much complexity and so much to consider. It is a whole other book!

An expert eye also protects you against becoming obsessive about tracking what you put into your body.* I'm careful to follow the data and evidence, but equally careful not to allow tracking my data to become obsessive** as this could have a negative effect on my mental health. It helps me that Dr Tam is also a very kind person and very approachable. I maintain that the people who you choose to support you on your fitness journey – even if it's the influencers or experts you choose to watch on YouTube or Instagram – must be kind and understanding (they can still make you work hard though). I will never forget Dr Tam's face when, feeling a bit jaded and hungover one day in my kitchen, I absent-mindedly leaned across the kitchen island, picked up a tube of squirty cream and gave myself two generous blasts from the nozzle straight into my mouth 'for breakfast'. There was a moment of appalled silence before she started to laugh. Then we had a talk.

* It is really important to be alert to conditions such as orthorexia – an unhealthy focus on what you put into your body. If tracking and monitoring become obsessive and lead to deprivation, that can damage your overall wellbeing – the opposite of what we're trying to achieve here.

** There are a number of eating-disorder helplines you can contact if you're in the UK and experiencing a time of crisis and would like to talk to somebody. This includes the National Centre for Eating Disorders Support Line (UK): 0845 838 2040 https://eating-disorders.org.uk.

Biohacking, STEM health, personalised healthcare – whatever you want to call it, and at whatever level you choose to embrace it (including, apparently, Epsom salts in a bath) – can be a game changer. One of the attractions for me is that it represents a move from a one-size-fits-all prescriptive approach to health and fitness that often played out as 'do this now or fail!' and left you crushingly disappointed when it didn't work. We're all way too individual for that to be effective.

If you can monitor what's going on, you can also be really focused when it comes to the changes you make. And as this area progresses, apps, sensors and tests will help to address some of the parts of the wellbeing jigsaw that have been overlooked. For example, increasingly researchers are considering the way our mental health determines the effectiveness of our immune system. You can already track your stress levels (through cortisol levels) and if you find an issue you can move to either bring down those levels, or boost your immune system – preferably both. Another thing this reinforces for me is the need to connect mind and body and to work equally hard on them both. So in the next chapter we'll look more closely at how we can intervene to calm our minds . . .

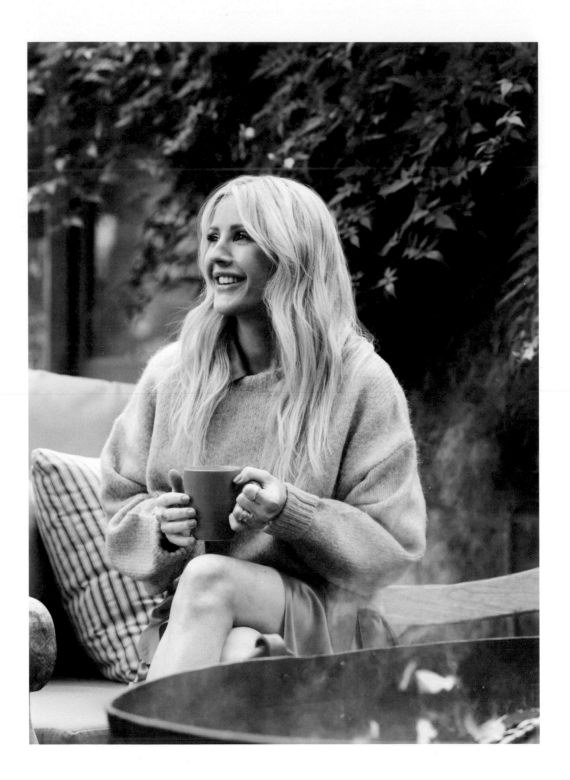

3

CALM YOUR MIND

'The nearer a WOMAN comes to a calm mind,
the closer SHE is to strength'
INSPIRED BY MARCUS AURELIUS, PHILOSOPER

I think a calm mind is one of the biggest luxuries on earth; I also think it's an absolute necessity. Yes, I know those two things seem contradictory, but I'm sticking with them. I call it a luxury because it seems to me to be the ultimate prize that we need to work really hard to attain. I'd rather have a calm mind than a new pair of shoes, a new car or even one of those massively expensive, very heavy scented candles with loads of wicks. It's such a gorgeous thing to know that you have that resource.

At the same time, it's really hard to buy yourself space in your head and to tune out the relentless onslaught of noise and negativity. A calm mind is actually something of a rarity. Meanwhile, we need it more than ever. In this chapter we'll talk about the steps you can take to protect yourself and achieve space from the stuff that disturbs your serenity – think of this stuff as the barrier to calm. We'll talk about the huge benefits of working hard to train your mind and share strategies that you can use to develop your ability to do this. Best of all, at this point in the book we get to hear from some of the incredible humans that have been so important in my fitness and wellbeing journey so far. We're starting in this chapter by talking to my friend Fearne Cotton, who has both actively pursued a more peaceful mind for herself and poured herself into opening up the conversation about mental health in the UK.

If this was easy to do, we'd all be doing it. But the fact is that the way we live now often works against. It can be difficult to attain much peace at all. Pressures of noise, urban living, stress, inequality, insecurity and unexpected happenings such as lockdowns all conspire to exert huge pressure on our mental wellbeing. At the same time, we also allow more pressure in – not least by allowing social media to call the shots; as we discussed earlier, there's a price to all that scrolling and you could be paying. I think it's critically important that we have strategies to help us navigate all of this, and that you put them to use as frequently as you would stretch after a workout.

One of the first things it can be useful to think about is your reaction when things go wrong. You're probably familiar with that saying 'shit happens'. Well, I prefer a longer version: 'shit happens, but it's your reaction that matters!' Because shit does happen, but it's often our reaction that casts the longer shadow. When I was younger, I reacted to a lot of situations with rage. Every time I reacted to something such as being dumped or arguing with a friend, anger would be my default.

The way we react is often down to lots of reasons we may not even be aware of. Some of us carry trauma from our childhood that affects how we react to situations years later. For some of us, it might be related to past relationships that weren't healthy or ended badly.

As you'll have seen already, I often try to connect the dots from how I'm feeling about a situation – fearful, rejected, insecure – to something that happened in my past. What I'm trying to work out is whether I am reacting to the situation that's happening right now in front of me, or whether my reaction is a throwback to something that's gone on before. I've learned to do this. Years ago, I would've just reacted angrily and forged ahead (only to spend hours agonising over whatever I'd said or done 48 hours later in a sort of shame-filled rebound moment, and for this to haunt me for the rest of my life). But reflecting – without judgement, but purely in order to establish whether my reaction is a spontaneous one or an emotional injury from the past – is really worth my time. As we know, positive change comes from understanding yourself better. I guess this monitoring is a bit like one of the bio-hacks we discussed in the previous chapter. Let's call it an emo-hack (as in emotional). And like its bio-hack cousin, time spent now will reap dividends as you progress.

Next time you react to something in a way that might seem out of sorts or even over the top, pause for a second to think about the real roots of your response. Some of us hold on to old battles, finding it hard to forgive, or some of us feel left out or hard done by and bring that to every argument and situation that follows.

In my case, getting over exes has always been particularly hard, because rejection is a bit of a trigger for me. I also struggle with the feeling of shame. Several years ago, I had a brief relationship that wasn't particularly serious, before I met somebody else who I decided I liked more. On reflection, this was a fairly normal, twentysomething situation. But because I'm in the public eye it became a story in the press. My actions and motivation were turned over in the press again and again. Of course, I wasn't permitted to tell my side of the story or even to make the point that as you fall in and out of romantic relationships in your late adolescence, not all of them work out! Hold the front page; what a shocker! The narrative was drawn and I was cast as a heartless bitch (one of the few roles available for young female pop stars at the time). Today we would say that I was slut-shamed and perhaps a few more people would have seen it from my point of view (we live in hope!). But back then, amid the slut-shaming and gossip, I felt the panic of my early twenties creep back. That feeling of being humiliated and judged haunted me for years, and it still does now from time to time.

You might think that's an extreme example and it probably is. But the common thread running through all of these emotions – shame, rejection – is that some of us are highly impacted if we feel we are not liked. And so many of my friends, who haven't been subjected to slut-shaming in the national press, tell me they are also gripped by this fear. It seems the playground dynamics where you are desperate to be liked and fit in stay with many of us for a long time, tragically sometimes all of our lives.

Perhaps you've felt it within your family? I don't think that feeling ever really leaves us. I've learned the hard way in the music industry that you're either liked or disliked, with rarely anything in between. And sometimes you can swing from one extreme to the other in the space of about an hour!

My advice is to try and avoid expending any energy on why you've fallen out of favour with anybody except those closest to you – it's too exhausting, too random – and focus on your reaction to it. Obviously the best reaction is to give zero fucks. But come on, that's pretty hard after you've been conditioned your whole life to try and please everybody – as many of us have. But I will take any grade of that; even giving fewer fucks than you did last time should be chalked up as a victory!

The next thing to do is to remove pressure from yourself to react at all, at least in the immediate sense. Of course, I still get stressed about work or anxious about stuff in my personal life, but I've learned not to react too quickly. A good exercise is to name the emotions that follow a bust-up (again, probably best to do it in your head, not out loud). It might take a little while and it may feel odd not to be releasing all of that reactionary energy as you usually would. But strap yourself into that rollercoaster and stay with the lows, the bends and turns. See how you feel when the rollercoaster stops. It can be uncomfortable to do this, and even painful, but it buys you time and gives you the opportunity to draw on rational thought processes, rather than reactionary instincts.

These days, instead of reacting, I tend to put my headphones on and do some meditation or go for a run. If I'm playing the long game and I need more time, I take myself off social media for a few days. This gives my emotions some time to settle and my mind time to process what's happened and work out what I should do next. And remember, I might choose to do nothing and that is a perfectly valid reaction, too.

The hangxiety: when a hangover destroys your calm

If you drink alcohol there's a high chance you've experienced a lot of emotional turbulence and anxiety the day after a big night out. Not everybody is impacted in this way, but it's so common a phenomenon that it now has a name: 'hangxiety' i.e. the chronic anxiety that comes with a hangover. I know I've experienced it many times and it always feels so unfair. How can you go from feeling on top of the world (or at least on top of the table you last remember dancing on) and giving your entire life story to the Uber driver (despite them not asking for it and being hilarious – um, at least I thought I was) on the way home, to being gripped by an anxiety so intense, you want to hide under the duvet. Cue endless WhatsApp messages to friends to try and gain reassurances that you didn't offend anybody, and manic scrolling to try and find clues from social media.

It turns out scientists are also interested in hangxiety and have developed a series of theories as to why it happens. There are some fascinating pieces out there if you look up hangxiety online, but this is my understanding of what happens. Essentially alcohol is a sedative that has an effect on our brain in a variety of ways. When it comes to a stonking attack of hangxiety, the most important one of these brain pathways is the gamma aminobutyric acid pathway, or GABA pathway. Alcohol activates the GABA activity in the brain (the stuff GABA is involved with includes motor control, memory and anxiety) sending chemical messages through the central nervous system that end up calming the brain and making fewer neurons fire, which is why you get that nice chill after a couple of drinks.

But then you carry on (because that's just what we do) and what starts to happen is the brain blocks the glutamate receptors, making us even less anxious ('I'm certain this

dancing is sensational, yep, I'm the best dancer in the room').
As the night wears on, your poor brain does its best to balance
this crazy mix of brain chemicals and reassert some control.
Your body is now on a mission to bring your GABA levels
back down to earth, and switch your glutamate back up.
Unfortunately, this leads to the jitteriness and sometimes
panicky feelings we now know as hangxiety.

I'm saying this, not because I want to put a downer on
your next Christmas party, or your best friend's wedding, but
because the more we understand that we feel like this because
of chemical responses and neurological responses, the more
certain we can be that it's not because we're terrible people
and we can rationalise quicker when it happens. When it comes
to drinking alcohol, I find that better understanding the effects
of drinking too much and how that might throw my body out of
balance has led me to become a much more mindful drinker.
I really do enjoy the drinks I do have, but I try not to overdo it!
(If you are struggling with alcohol or drugs please speak to
your GP as soon as possible. NHS online has a list of resources
and helpline numbers you can contact www.nhs.uk/live-well/
alcohol-support/)

Here are three things to remember when your mind is full of turbulence:

'Do not trust the way you see yourself
Do not create assumptions about others
Wait until you feel better to make final decisions
that have long-term effects'

YUNG PUEBLO, POET AND ACTIVIST

Pottering Time . . .

I want to talk a little bit about emotional time management. As we've already discussed, I think it's worth giving time to understanding your feelings more deeply. But I can also recognise when someone is busying themselves to the point where they're never alone with their own thoughts. After all, it can be all too easy to bury uncomfortable thoughts if we're constantly on the go, surrounded by others with no time left to think. The reason why that isn't terribly helpful is because, as we've already discussed, unresolved thoughts and issues have a way of sticking around, dominating your thoughts and sort of pushing calm and serenity out.

People who always need to be with others, for example, are often the people who never want to leave the party. From the outside they look fun and extrovert, but sometimes there's something else going on.

I was one of those people for a while during my twenties. The highs of being on stage are immense and hugely addictive. But when I came off stage and the highs weren't there, I missed them and wanted to fill that void. At the same time, I avoided big crowds and after-parties because of social anxiety – so I was a real mess, basically. There are lots of versions of this scenario – the person who always wants to go out drinking after work, or the person who fills their diary up to the point they rush from one social event to the next. If this sounds like you, take a step back and ask yourself why you're doing this.

Making a little chunk of time each day or each week where you're on your own and enjoying your own company, whether it's at the gym or pottering at home, will give you time to process your thoughts, fears and emotions. This involves taking some time alone each day and getting used to being on your own (and enjoying it!). One of the things I heard a lot during the pandemic and lockdowns was the totally understandable gripe that with everyone at home (including home schooling for the kids) there was 'no space'. What we often meant by that was not just a lack of physical space (although that, too) but primarily a lack of mental space.

Being OK with being alone also means that when you do choose to spend time with people – whether that's a boyfriend, girlfriend, friends or colleagues – you pick good people who add to your life and make you happy. I went through times where I was a serial monogamist, out of one long-term relationship and then into the next: I was always with somebody. Those people weren't always adding to my life or making me happy – and I definitely wasn't making them happy in return. I didn't always feel particularly healed in my twenties, so I would choose people who I could continue to be unhealed with. I could carry on with whatever toxic behaviour I happened to be choosing at the time, like working too hard, because in effect they allowed me to get away with it. Meanwhile, I kept up this façade of a happy, confident woman.

Looking back, I think I attracted friends who liked the person I was pretending to be. I don't want to put too much on this. For most people, their twenties can be a tough decade because there is so much to untangle emotionally. I still had a huge amount of fun, too, but deep down was I happy? I don't think so. Because of my experience, it has become really important to me to avoid making others responsible for your happiness. Nobody else is your happiness-maker. We also need to ask ourselves, am I with this person because they make me happy and add something to my life? Or am I with this person because I don't want to be lonely?

It took me a long time to get to the place I am in now, where I'm absolutely fine if Caspar has to go away for work, or if I don't have plans on a Saturday night. Because now I know I'm fine on my own. In fact, I'm better than fine. I'm absolutely happy and content.

The power of friendships

Despite the importance of learning to be OK on your own, having good friendships and nurturing them is essential for your wellbeing, too.

The quality (not quantity) of our relationships with those around us plays such an important role in our health. Humans are social animals and countless studies show that one of the best predictors for longevity and good health is the strength of our social connections. Many of us now maintain our friendships online, which has merits and was something of a life saver during Covid-19, but the power of touch, of hugs, of hearing somebody's voice on the phone and laughing together until you cry can't be underestimated. My mum was very tactile and was always giving us hugs, so now I'm a real hugger. When I'm away from Caspar, hugs are the things I miss most.

'Attributes of a good friend:

They feel like home

They are honest with you

They remind you of your power

They support you in your healing

They have a rejuvenating presence

They hold a vision of your success

They support you in new adventures

They lift you up with joy and laughter

They bring out the best version of you'

YUNG PUEBLO

I bloody love my friends. I really do. This is a change for me. I mean, I always loved them, but I used to be more standoffish. In my twenties I lived in my head quite a lot. I was fiercely independent and I didn't always turn to friends when I needed them. But now I'm always on their case. Before coronavirus, so much of my job involved networking, socialising and partying, and I met different people all the time, who flitted in and out of my life. But during lockdown it was my oldest friends I called the most. As the saying goes, when life gets tough, you find out who you want your friends to be.

Right at the start of my career, I asked my best friend Hannah from university to come and work with me and she's on my management team to this day. I remember meeting Hannah at university and thinking she was far too pretty and cool to be associated with the likes of me, shuffling about in flares with a guitar case. That's what it's like when you're a teenager, right? But I quickly realised she's totally bonkers and we've been best friends ever since. Another best friend is my make-up artist, Lucy, and another my stylist, Nathan (who we met briefly in Chapter 1 when he launched one his very gentle and intuitive truth bombs).

Although I wouldn't have it any other way, it can be quite tricky working with your friends. Essentially, I'm their boss, so that can add a layer of awkwardness. If I ever need to tell them to do things a different way, it's hard to know whether to approach them with that as a friend or a boss. And if work is really busy and Hannah is texting me a lot and asking me to 'OK' stuff like I'm Alan Sugar or something, every now and then I'll say, 'Can you text me as a friend because I'm missing that side of things?' Fortunately she knows what I'm on about.

Most of my very close friends come from the time before I was famous, but I still seek out positive, funny and interesting people, and I've met a lot of great people through Caspar. Something that absolutely fascinated me about him when we met was the sheer amount of incredible women he surrounded himself with. A testament to him, I guess.

I've also made friends in my industry who are just fascinating human beings. Some are supremely intelligent artists, writers, fashion people or critics, and I'm proud to know them. But you know what? It's not the same as being able to fart in front of them like I would with my schoolfriends. I'm not sure how this last paragraph converts into a bit of advice. Perhaps it's this: make sure you've got friends you can fart in front of. (They'll appreciate that!)

A word on families

Family relationships can be incredibly complex and complicated, as many people know. Conversely, if you're very close to your parents or siblings and have a straightforward relationship with them, it can be difficult to understand those who don't. But do try. Perhaps you have a friend or a colleague who doesn't speak to certain family members or goes for long periods without seeing or speaking to them. So many people are in this position and I think it should be talked about more. There's so much more we could say on this topic – again, it's another whole book – but I do I think the idea that you should be best friends with your whole family, no matter what, is fundamentally flawed. If there's somebody in your family who is making you feel like shit, or is gaslighting you, whether they know they're doing it or not, then it's OK not to have them as a central figure in your life and I don't think you should feel guilty about it. I really believe that. And it's probably why my non-familial friendships are doubly important to me. That's not to say that any family falling-out is irreparable, as I'm a firm believer that, with time, most things can be resolved.

'The deepest friendships reveal themselves during moments of crisis. When your world is shaken, they stand and face the storm with you. When things look dim, they bring their light to remind you that better days are coming. When you feel challenged, they help you see your power.'

YUNG PUEBLO

I want you to try exercising a new power. It's the power of saying 'no' sometimes.

I discovered it about four years ago, as I approached the age of thirty. I'm not sure where it had been hiding, but this secret power has become one of the most important ways I achieve calm and balance in my life today. As we've already seen in the previous chapters, I was working too hard before that to really find out who I was. As I approached thirty, I realised what I was doing. I was setting myself on fire to keep everyone else warm. Obviously, I mean this metaphorically. I have never literally set myself on fire and nobody has asked me to. But there's a great chance you have also done this at points in your life. And you only really stop when you realise the power of saying 'no'.

I'm so grateful that I got to a point of understanding where I realised how much of an investment it would be to take a step back for a while and take on less work. When I came to this realisation, the quality of everything improved and I felt like I could give a better version of myself, even if I seemed like I had moved slightly under the radar as an artist. I just liked myself better and I liked my art more. Learning to say no is really about learning to know your self-worth. When you say yes to absolutely everything – whether that's in your career, in relationships, with friends, or with your family – you're doing it at the expense of your own time and your own happiness and sense of calm. What you're really saying is that you don't matter.

That's why I say you are setting yourself on fire to keep everyone else warm.

In the case of work, our inability to say 'no' is often rooted in the Impostor Syndrome we talked about earlier in this book. Because you don't feel legitimate, you fear that if you say no to one opportunity, others won't come your way. But if you're good at what you do and work hard, of course they will come back. You're the kween! And you'll be healthier, happier, more rested and better at what you do for the break. That's a good trade-off for saying 'no' occasionally. Oh, and you don't have to be rude: if you're nervous of that, just say 'no, thank you'.

Nowadays, I prioritise exercise and making good food because I know how epic it makes me feel, and I know that will help me to think clearly when I'm writing and to perform when I'm on stage. Don't get me wrong, sometimes a lack of clarity and chaos, and maybe a few drinks, is required to write songs. But generally, I like to feel calm and peaceful, especially in the ever-changing, increasingly mad world we find ourselves living in.

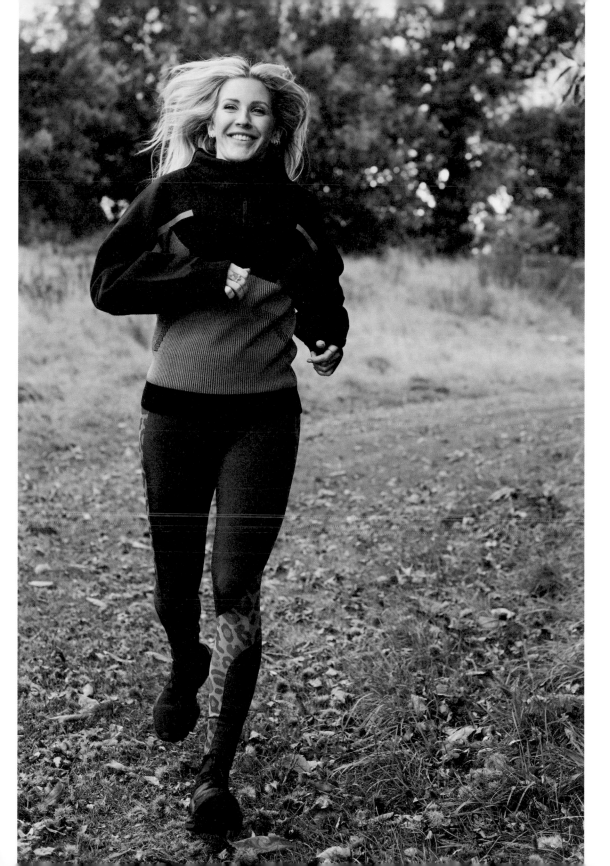

Meet . . . FEARNE COTTON

Fearne is a TV, radio and podcast presenter, and a dear friend of mine who I met very early on in my career. I've always loved her approach to life, work and wellness, but more than anything I love her kindness and honesty.

Ellie: Do you remember when we first met?

> **Fearne:** 'I remember you first walking into the Live Lounge at Radio 1 many pop moons ago. Bobble hat bouncing along as you strode, guitar in hand, towards the mic. I had yet to hear your voice live, so I was floored by your ethereal acoustic version of "Starry Eyed". You later revealed you were so nervous doing that first Live Lounge, yet no one would have known.
>
> 'You've been a class act from day one and brought to the table something entirely fresh and exciting. I love that you've always done things your own way.'

Ellie: Do you think our approaches to life, stress and wellbeing are fairly similar?

> **Fearne:** 'Due to our weird jobs and our respective stumbling through life in the public eye, I think we have naturally fallen into a similar rhythm when it comes to looking after ourselves. I think you realise early on in this industry that you can easily get burned out and there is always another job to be done if you don't say no.'

Ellie: How did you find the pressure of becoming famous?

> **Fearne:** 'The outside pressure can be quite intense, as your every move is scrutinised and judged, so unless you learn coping mechanisms your sanity is on the line. But you had a much quicker and more extreme ascent in your career than I did, so in ways I

was lucky to gradually get used to the pressures from a young age, yet never to the gargantuan global level you have dealt with. I think we both love to keep active and to ponder life's bigger questions. I'm not sure I'll ever be as badass at boxing as you, but I'm always inspired by your work and workout ethic.'

Ellie: How have you learned to deal with stress?

Fearne: 'At times I'm good at letting go and seeing the bigger picture. But more often than not, I go through a process where I feel myriad emotions and then reach an outcome. It'll often start with stress or anger and then lead to shame or sorrow and eventually arrive at peace and acceptance. As I get more dedicated to living in a peaceful way, the process gets quicker.'

Ellie: What sort of things do you do when you start to feel overwhelmed?

Fearne: 'They are all rather obvious, but easily overlooked when you're rushing through life. I love to walk and run and be in nature. The more we understand our own individual and collective connection to nature, the bigger chance we have of finding peace. Nature works harmoniously and grows without a fight or struggle. Plants bloom, then die and then the cycle starts over again. Often in the modern world we want to keep pushing and quickening the speed at which we live. Nature tells us again and again that we need to rest, reset and pause. We can always look to nature for the answers.'

Ellie: How about exercise?

Fearne: 'I love yoga for calming down my own hyper nervous system and also meditating using guided mediations. Music has always been a great tonic for me too and usually helps me align with what I'm feeling on a much deeper level.'

Ellie: I learned a lot of this stuff the hard way. Is that something you can relate to?

> *Fearne:* 'Yes, but I wouldn't change that. I used to burn out regularly and feel very low due to my lack of reserves, energy and time. Now I'm much better at setting boundaries as to what I want to do and don't. I've learned to take the "shoulds" out of my life and try to work with what I want to do. It might sound incredibly selfish, but it really doesn't have to be. When we really listen to our intuition it often wants to help others, be of service and help the ripple effect of joy to continue rolling on.'

Ellie: Have you ever struggled with your emotional health?

> *Fearne:* 'I hit a big patch of depression in my late twenties/early thirties and felt floored by how different the world looked to me through a new pitch-black lens. My values were considerably different from how they stand today as I placed importance on things that don't matter to me at all today.'

Ellie: How did you overcome that?

> *Fearne:* 'I pressed reset and started over again, learning to eradicate shame and embarrassment and to cultivate peace and acceptance of myself. Also, talking to others about the parts of me that I thought alienated me gave me such relief. I realised that those parts of me are in fact the bits that connect me to others the most. Depression and panic attacks felt heavy and secret and not something to share and shout about, but now they are some of my favourite things to talk about. Self-acceptance is vastly underrated. I'm over trying to be someone else and buying new stuff to enhance who I think I should be, and am fully accepting of the slightly scruffy, paradoxically insanely organised, flawed, energetic, enthusiastic, complicated woman that I am.'

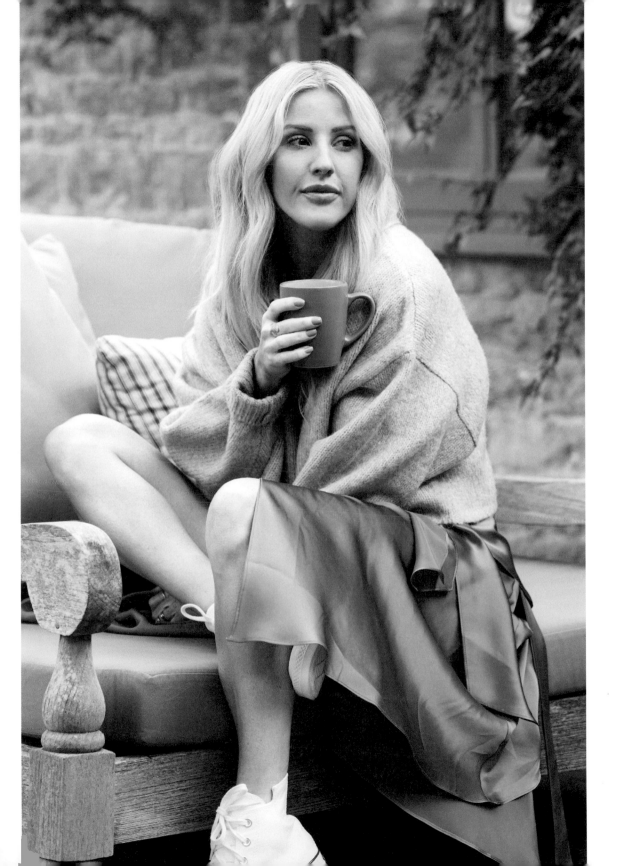

Here are some other ways to feel happier and more positive:

GET OUTSIDE

Researchers from the Finnish Forest Research Institute found that people feel psychologically restored after just 15 minutes of sitting outside in either a park or forest. Wherever you live, even if it's in a city, go and find some green space and sit in it for a while. When I'm in London I'll often head for a walk or a jog around my nearest park. This is about using your time restoratively, and you can't do that if you're on your phone. Leave it behind, or keep it in your pocket. And remember there's no such thing as bad weather – only bad clothing – so even on the days it's wet, windy or rainy, wrap up warm and get outside. (Plus if you live in the UK and you're avoiding rain and wind you're not going to get out much).

GARDEN FOR YOUR MENTAL HEALTH

The research between growing plants and beneficial mental health seems to be sprouting from every academic institution. One report from the King's Fund found that gardening can help reduce depression and anxiety. Another, from the University of Exeter and the Royal Horticultural Society, found that the health and wellbeing benefits of gardening were similar to living in the richest part of the country. The study also found that people who regularly spend time in their gardens were significantly more likely to be physically active and have higher psychological wellbeing than those who don't. So plant whatever is in season, or get pottering or pruning. (If it's coming into winter and nothing is really growing, get out and tidy.) Just 10 minutes a day will help reduce stress and make you feel better. If you live in a flat and have a balcony or a windowsill, you can still make the most of the space you have through container gardening, growing herbs or other plants. Or put your name down for an allotment; there are over 300,000 in the UK.

LISTEN TO MUSIC

This is a classic piece of advice, but it works. The health benefits of this are long and proven. Listening to music can help to improve mood, overall wellbeing, relaxation and happiness levels, as well as reducing stress and anxiety, helping us to regulate and make sense of our emotions. It can even help with easing pain, boosting brain power and improving memory. A study published in the journal *Music & Science* also found that listening to music increases our empathy and fosters a sense of connection in the listener.

I don't really listen to pop music on my days off, because I can't help making it about work and end up analysing the lyrics and the notes of the music. I'm obsessed with the art of pop music and the formulas behind it. But to me that is work. So when I want to switch off I listen to a lot of classical music. There's something so profound about classical music, the pureness of it and the visceral feelings you get when you listen to a live orchestra. It affects me on such a deep level. It often gives me goosebumps. If you have never listened to classical music but feel like you want a change, Radio 3 and Classic FM are good places to start, or simply select a classical playlist on a streaming platform.

WRITE IT OUT TO CLEAR YOUR HEAD

'Journalling', as the practice of writing everything down has become known, makes me think of little Victorian ladies for some reason. I suppose it's also a bit of a wellbeing cliché, but it's very popular and that's probably because it works! Writing down all your thoughts, however random, has the benefit of clearing them out of your head so they don't have to spin around in there day and night. You can jot down anything from anxieties and worries to everyday to-do lists. If you don't process this stuff, as we know to our cost, it can end up lodged in your head, leaving you feeling anxious and overwhelmed.

When a worry, thought or chore is written down, the pressure is somehow released from it.

You could also jot down a list of things you are grateful for. Studies show gratitude reduces toxic emotions like envy and resentment. It can also increase empathy, help with sleep and improve self-esteem. Other studies show it can reduce our need to socially compare ourselves (as we've acknowledged, this is destructive) and improves our mental strength and resilience, making it easier to bounce back from stressful situations.

I have always felt that I put all my thoughts and fears into songs, which is maybe why I haven't 'journalled' that much myself. But writing about the benefits really makes me want to do it! I do sometimes like to write essays on topics that interest me. I don't necessarily do anything with them, although some have been published, but I love putting pen to paper and getting down all the thoughts that whirl around my head in a narrative form. If you are particularly affected by something in the world, perhaps climate change, or the fact that teachers or nurses aren't paid enough, it can be really beneficial to write about it, because it then encourages you to gather more information about that subject; and as we know, knowledge is power!

PRIORITISE YOUR SLEEP

Full disclosure: I'm a terrible sleeper. There are nights when I lie awake, distracted by a noise outside my house, or a niggling thought that's been bothering me for a while. Sometimes I think about something I said to someone YEARS ago – 'maybe I offended them' – or my mind drifts to whether a certain song could have had a different melody. So, while I'm not a good sleeper, nor a sleep expert, there are certain things I've learned over the years that help me to sleep better. The first is to prioritise your sleep like you do your workouts or your diet. That means getting a little pre-bed routine in place, such as having a bath using some nice bath oils and reading a book in there.

Take a technology break an hour before bed and read instead. Some people can go to sleep minutes after scrolling through social media, and if I'm in the right frame of mind, I can too. But if I'm worried or anxious about something, doing that means I'll stay awake worrying about whatever I've seen on there. Or I'll wake up early and do the same as well. I remember vividly a few months ago being in a really nice, sleepy, happy state, ready for a good sleep, then without thinking I opened Instagram and saw something that made my blood boil. It caused a domino effect: I slept really badly for the entire week and felt off my game at a live performance.

Moving your body before sleep also helps. We're not talking a pre-bed HIIT class (that will energise you; we need you to settle) but a simple Pilates or yoga session will help quieten your mind. Good sleep is so important. Studies show that poor sleep raises our risk of catching a cold by suppressing our immune system, it reduces motivation, concentration, slows down our reaction times and increases our appetite by switching on our 'hunger hormones' and dialling down our satiety ones, so we never feel full and are more likely to crave sugar. More seriously, poor sleep over time can also raise our risk of diseases like diabetes, depression and heart disease. Sleep is one of the most powerful performance enhancers and mood boosters there is, so take some time to work out how to improve your sleep routine.

If you have the ability, everyone should track their sleep – start with the number of hours and how refreshed you feel in the morning, then try changing up your pre-bed routine: 10 minutes of meditation, a warm shower or bath, half an hour of reading a book. I use different sleep monitors, or 'wearables' (see Chapter 2, 'Listen to Your Body') and have found tracking my sleep has led to one of the biggest positive changes to the rest of my life by helping me to improve quality and quantity. In turn, this has benefited my mood, my energy, my strength and my creativity.

I know I keep banging my drum here, but I really feel so

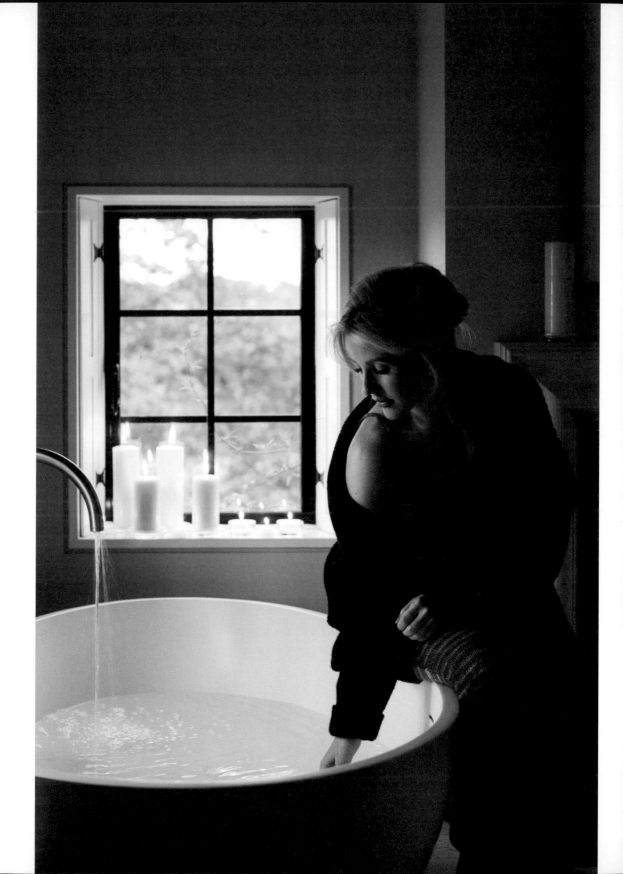

strongly that there needs to be more awareness around how good fitness is for your mental health. So much of the fitness conversation is around calories burned and muscles stretched, but I've found from personal experience that the muscle that benefits most from exercise is your brain. It stands to reason. When you move your body for any length of time – no matter how you do it – your brain releases dopamine and serotonin, which are the feel-good hormones responsible for regulating your mood. Exercise regularly and the serotonin levels in your brain will stay raised.

So the final top tip I can give you about attaining the luxurious necessity of a calm mind (which is also a happy mind) is to keep moving! Luckily, as we move on through the book, you are going to find lots of ways to make that happen. In Chapter 6 I'm going to zero in on the importance of movement (there I go again!) and explain how all the different types of exercise I've tried have helped boost my mood and quieten any anxiety. I know I'm definitely not the only one obsessed with movement as the key to mental as well as physical health – phew! Catie Miller, a brilliant teacher of 'Barre', and a source of constant inspiration to me, explains more in both Chapters 6 and 7 through her specially devised barre workouts. In fact, I'm going to end this chapter with her very wise words:

'You can only control what you can control. So whether it's work, illness, divorce, finances, family, or something else entirely that is causing you stress, remember that all of us will go through periods of stress and there's often little we can do about it, other than to adapt to what's happening and then find the tools to feel safe. For me, movement is key and it's something that has carried me through many of life's upheavals.'

CATIE MILLER, BARRE TEACHER

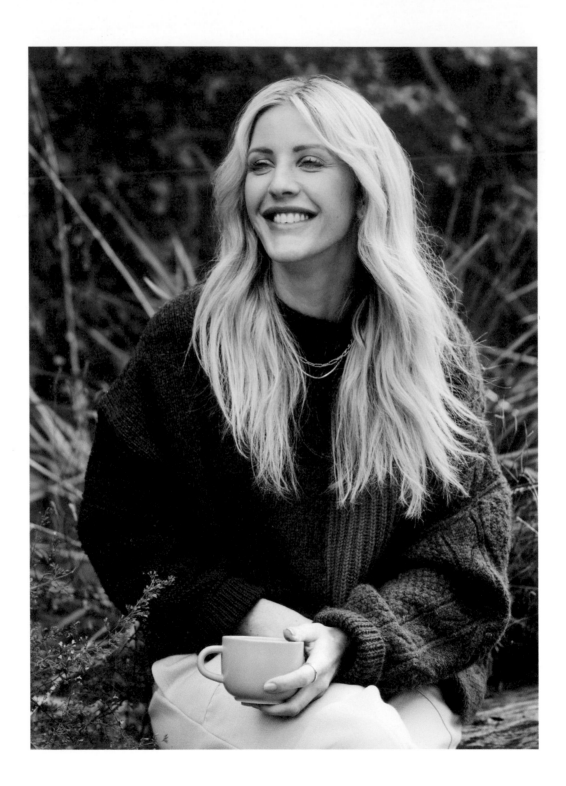

4 NOURISH YOUR BODY

'Every time you eat is an opportunity to nourish your body'

ANON

I think food should be joyful. It's as simple as that. For complex reasons (some of which we'll touch on in this chapter) food is often demonised. I don't mean we push our trolleys around the supermarket waving our fists at packets of biscuits, but somewhere along the process of feeding ourselves, it can get fraught. I don't think terms like 'clean eating' have been helpful (and we'll discuss this later with nutritionist Pixie Turner). When you have 'clean' food, by definition you also characterise everything else as 'dirty'. Meanwhile, the more obsessive you get over food, the more you lose sight of its pleasures.

For me, one of the joys of living is to have a takeaway with friends. But I know if I had them all the time, it wouldn't be enjoyable. The key is that I see these takeouts with friends as occasions. If I did it every day or multiple times a week, I would not feel good about myself (also I'd really worry about the packaging as I'm a bit of a tree hugger).

On that note – I actually I think there's a close relationship between thinking of food from a fitness standpoint and as an environmental campaigner. The latter makes me aware that the planet can't sustain our food habits. Processed, fast food and foods with lots of sugar in them often have a heavy impact on the planet. A 2018 study found that in the UK, the chocolate industry is responsible for two million metric tons of carbon dioxide (CO_2) emissions. That's because you have to factor in all the cocoa, milk, manufacturing and shipping involved – a lot of resources and a lot of energy means a lot of carbon is produced. Other studies show that meat eaters have twice the carbon footprint of those who follow a plant-based diet. (This has a lot to do with cow farts, but I don't want to sound like I'm obsessed with flatulence, so I'll leave that explanation for another time!)

The point for me is that foods with greater impact on health and the planet are often the ones we associate with joy. And if we treat them, well, like treats, that not only enhances our enjoyment when we have them, but it takes the pressure off. If we eat party foods all day long, our bodies and the planet can't handle it. There's a very clever UK academic, Professor Tim Lang, who has written many books, including his most recent, *Feeding Britain: our food problems and how to fix them*, and he wraps this up in a simple bit of advice, 'Have feast day foods only on feast days.' I love this, and although Prof. Lang is talking principally about the environmental effect of foods with big impacts, I think it's great advice that translates to a health context, too.

As I've done elsewhere in this book, I'm going to be as honest as I can about my own experiences. And to be completely honest, in the past I've had a complex relationship with food. In common with many, I developed some strange assumptions (remember, it's all in the mind!). For instance, at times I've pretty much existed on sugar, because I assumed it was OK to do that while I was running it all off in the gym. Spoiler: it isn't OK.

I've also tried many different types of diet. Most recently I tried keto – the ketogenic diet, which is a very low-carb and high-fat diet that is similar to the Atkins diet (that's the one everyone did in the 1990s). Replacing carbs with fat is supposed to put your body into a metabolic state called 'ketosis', which is when fat burning occurs. But I've started eating carbs again recently because I missed them, and I'm feeling more comfortable eating them. Like exercise, I try to stay flexible about the way I eat; I like trying new things. I sometimes go too far in one direction or the other, but overall I strive to keep things balanced and ultimately nourishing. I also listen closely to my body.

It's such a cliché, but you have to take a balanced approach to food. If you have a takeaway one night, bloody enjoy it and don't feel guilty, but the next day be more mindful about what you eat (note: not obsessive). If you feel that you're gaining weight – before making a huge change, and trying an extreme diet suddenly – first try smaller changes. This could be having a few big salads for dinner a couple of nights a week (see Chapter 8 for some ideas) or try swapping out chips or rice for vegetables. This is about being aware of what you're eating, because this is the nourishment that provides fuel for your life, rather than being obsessive, which frankly lacks long-term planning (sorry to sound like a financial advisor, but we do have to think ahead!). Oh, and always remember going to the supermarket when you're hungry NEVER works out. (Don't blame me if you get home with nineteen bags of jelly based confectionery and three cream cakes.)

My journey with food

Growing up, I ate rapidly and gravitated towards sugar. Breakfast times really stand out in my memory. There were usually about four different types of cereal on offer, ranging from the worthy to the ones absolutely dripping in sugar.

I would grab my cereal, then proceeded to pour a lot of very cold milk on top and eat it so quickly my stomach would hurt. When you are one of four kids – I have one older sister, one younger sister and a younger brother – this is how breakfasts are. You absolutely do not want to be the one left with the most boring cereal (i.e. the least sugary). In fact, I often used to attempt to hide the 'best' one from my siblings, to guarantee my bowl. I would also shovel peas onto my poor brother's plate when he wasn't looking. I detested them – and most other green foods, come to think of it. The only green I was in favour of were brightly coloured green sweets.

Of course, like most kids, I was never really that conscious of what I was eating. I didn't make the connection between the food I was putting into my body and the way my body felt.

If I quickly ate a bowl of sugary cereal drenched in milk and then developed a stomach ache, I didn't connect the dots. The stomach ache was just a mystery of my body, like getting a headache or a cough. It was out of my control, or so I thought.

Looking back, pretty much all my meals were loaded with sugar. Sandwiches, crisps and a Penguin or Club bar for lunch; and tea would be anything from that classic 1980s childhood medley of fish fingers, chips and baked beans, to a shepherd's pie or Sunday roast. I remember some of my friends were quite envious of this diet – pretty standard for the time. They were raised more on organic vegetables, pulses and salads. Looking back, I probably felt quite sorry for them.

But it was sugar that had my heart (and my taste buds) The high-school tuck shop was my happy place, and I can still taste the lukewarm chocolate doughnuts at break time, oozing with some sort of unidentifiable but utterly delicious sweet brown gooey liquid.

Given that I sustained a perpetual sugar rush, it's little wonder that most of my school reports said things like 'Clever, gets the work done, but lacking in concentration and focus . . .'

At the age of fourteen, I watched a short documentary on how meat ended up on our plates. I was horrified. It sounds strange because Hereford is very much a farming community, but I had never really considered the backstory of anything I ate, never mind how animals got on my plate (yes, obviously I realised they were killed). Overnight, I went from a consumer of meat-and-two-veg to just the two veg. But as I didn't really like veg, I augmented it with that classic . . . toast. Being a vegetarian when you don't really like vegetables (or salads) is not very fulfilling. A bit later on, when I was a student and working as a part-time barmaid at a local pub that did great roast dinners, I existed almost entirely on potatoes and gravy. *face palm*

'Don't obsessively overthink every meal, just be a little bit more aware of what you're eating'

ELLIE

In common with many teenagers, this was also the beginning of a slightly complicated relationship with food that lasted into my mid-twenties. Unless you're lucky enough to develop a strong, sensible and balanced view of food early on, chances are you've experienced your own version of this story; whether it's about meat or sugar, alcohol or overeating, or controlling what you eat, it's shocking how many of us have a story of a difficult relationship with food. The reasons as to why that would be are complex, but I know we are not to blame.

I was lucky that I was able to repair this fractured relationship. It just took a long time. The key for me was making the connection between what I ate and how I felt. Our food choices can make the difference between feeling happy and sad and being productive or sluggish. They also play a major role in our overall health.

But as a teenager that didn't occur to me (and looking back there wasn't much education). So a lack of understanding and knowledge coincided with the fact that your teenage years and twenties are a time when image becomes everything. Being attractive to the opposite sex meant – in my teenage mind, at least – having 'decent boobs', barely any bottom (which was the fashion at the time; the opposite is now the case), being tanned, being skinny, but not too skinny, and somehow being skinny with big boobs. That's a kind of unattainable silhouette for many. Well, it certainly was for me, because I was kind of awkward looking; I was pale and freckly, and I definitely didn't have any boobs to write home about.

I knew how I wanted to look in my mind, and I thought I knew how I should look. But that didn't tally with what I saw in the mirror. All my bumps seemed to me to be in the wrong places.

Becoming a teenager meant becoming noticed and judged by the boys in our year*. Suddenly spots appeared, my hair got thinner and my weight began to fluctuate. I hated showing any flesh, so avoided fashion – at that point, tight crop tops and low-slung cargo pants – and became a 'grunger'. This meant dressing as much like my male idols as possible and piercing as much as I could get away with. My body was obscured under gigantic hoodies and flared jeans, and completely hidden behind the guitar I carried.

By the time I reached sixth-form college as a late teen, I was experiencing excruciating stomach aches. After doing some research myself, I decided I most likely had IBS (irritable bowel syndrome) and eventually came to the conclusion it was probably to do with all the bread and wheat I was eating. But I was so committed to eating bread that I decided the stomach aches were worth it; not realising I was probably causing more and more problems for my poor gut. Looking back now, that is a very strange commitment. I was more committed to bread than my health. Wow!

* In recent times there has been open discussion and dialogue about this type of peer to peer judging between boys and girls at school. The Everyone's Invited platform disclosed some truly awful examples of the pressure exerted on young women at schools in the UK around appearance and sex. I really welcome the fact that we're beginning to have honest dialogue about abuse towards women, girls and marginalised genders that has become almost normalised, but we must focus on solutions. In my Pass the Mic series that I host on my Instagram I interviewed an amazing man, Dr Jackson Katz. He is an author, with a PhD in cultural studies and education, on gender, race and violence and he runs education programmes that tackle these issues head on. I really recommend any of his writing or his TED Talk if you want to know more.

Eating on tour

By the time I was in my twenties, I was on the road being a full-time pop star. Some people in the music industry can't remember much at all about their touring years (especially from the 1960s and 70s!). They're hazy about who they married, never mind what they ate. But I know exactly what my diet was like on tour because I always had exactly the same thing: salad, side of fries and sweets to follow. This was my tour-bus diet and my hotel room-service diet . . . for years. Now remember, during this time I went to places that are famous for cuisine. I went to the epicentres of vegetarian food cultures, lands where the really pricey fruits that we import grow right there on trees, where the food culture dates back to the dawn of civilization. I could have been like the late great Anthony Bourdain*, savouring this culinary odyssey, but no, 'can I have a big salad and a side of fries please?'

The stomach aches got worse. I always give my stage performances everything. I expend every bit of energy I have, so when I came off-stage I was ravenous and would wolf down my salad 'n' chips. It was a fear that I would not be able to maintain my energetic performances on stage that made me decide to change the way I approached food. If I couldn't control touring (and this is the same as if you work away from home a lot in any job), I could try and make it accommodate me. Elsewhere in this book, I talk about setting fire to yourself to keep everyone else warm (again, metaphorically). My hang-ups about food, which involved negative self-image, a need for sugar, obsessive behaviour (always eating the same thing) and a lack of connection, had collided with this idea of sacrificing myself to put on a show.

I started to make some changes. Being the frontwoman has many drawbacks, but you are also ultimately your own boss.

* The US chef and writer who made his name with a brilliant exposé about working in restaurants, *Kitchen Confidential*, and went on to tour the world trying food in the TV show Parts Unknown.

And that meant I could put a few rules in place about catering to help myself out. If the typical caricature of a spoiled celebrity involves a rider where blue M&Ms must be removed, I decided mine would be about fruit platters and rice cakes. I know I can't eat for 3 hours before I sing, so on a performance day I would sustain myself with a small handful of blueberries or raspberries (later on I realised, working with experts like Pixie, who you'll meet shortly, that this wasn't quite right. But I was trying.)

After the show, I would go to my dressing room, and there were always people to hang out with. Now I would make sure there were lots of chopped vegetables, hummus and berries laid out, too. I like being able to grab and dip and eat quick and healthy filling food while talking to people. I also had a brilliant vegan chef who would come on tour with me and she would make these huge, amazing vegan salads or vegan pizzas. She even brought a little stove on tour and would make vegan Southern Fried Chicken.

I don't know if you've ever been on a tour bus with a load of blokes, but it's not very glamorous (no offence, guys!). The musicians seemed to entirely exist on crisps and pizzas. I still wanted to join in occasionally – remember 'treat food' (see page 85) – but I also introduced a smoothie bar on the bus, bringing a blender and loads of fruit and veg, and green powders and protein.

These were big changes for me. They weren't perfect – you might remember in Chapter 2 when I started monitoring my glucose it transpired that my smoothie habit was to blame for spikes in insulin levels, and I had to modify my recipes. But these changes were part of an evolving connection I was making to how I nourished myself and how I felt.

You will have your own food history and it may be even more complex and even more emotive. Or if you're lucky, you may have a wonderful functioning relationship with nutrition. Good for you. But in my experience, almost everyone can benefit from the perspective of a very good nutritionist. So for the next part of this chapter, I'm going to speak to Pixie Turner.

Meet . . . PIXIE TURNER

Pixie is a qualified nutritionist and ACT therapist specialising in intuitive eating, disordered eating and body image.

Ellie: What's your food ethos?

> **Pixie:** 'When it comes to food, it's simple: it's there to be enjoyed. Eating isn't a choice, like deciding whether to run or do yoga. It's something we all need to do, every single day. So it should be as enjoyable an experience as possible. Yet all too often it seems to be wrapped up in guilt, shame and rules. I often think as a society we have overcomplicated things.'

Ellie: In what way?

> **Pixie:** 'I'll give you an anecdote from my early twenties. On my twenty-second birthday, and in the throes of my interest in "clean eating", my mother presented me with a raw, vegan birthday cake, because she knew that was a good way to get me to eat cake. At the time I desperately convinced myself that I was enjoying it, but I picked at it miserably, not wanting to upset my family – who didn't like it – or waste an expensive cake either. Looking back, what I should have done was request a gloriously gooey chocolate fudge cake and just enjoyed it. That birthday was a real light-bulb moment for me and soon after that I went into nutrition as a career.'

Ellie: Why were you so hung up on food back then?

> **Pixie:** 'Three years earlier, aged nineteen, I had a bit of a health scare with my cholesterol levels. My doctor said it could be partly genetic, partly lifestyle. I was at university, studying biochemistry, and my doctor said that I should go away and see how things were within a year and if they were no better, I might

have to take medication for life. I decided to see if I could help myself and so I did what a lot of us do in these situations – I turned to Dr Google.'

Ellie: When was this?

Pixie: 'This was in 2012 when various wellness bloggers, both here and in Australia, were popping up all over Instagram to talk about how they had healed themselves from a variety of ailments through food. It was a time of peak food demonisation, when banishing so-called "bad" foods was at its height – sugar, dairy, carbs, alcohol, caffeine, you name it, you were told you should probably give it up if you wanted your diet to be "clean" so you could "glow with good health". It was all very intoxicating for somebody young and idealistic like me, whose intentions were good. I just wanted to be healthier after all, and this seemed like I was taking control of my health and nutrition. So in the place of all my old dietary staples there was a "clean diet" of mostly fresh fruits, raw vegetables, a few beans and seemingly little else.

'Certain beliefs quickly became mantras in that world: "Gluten damages your gut", "Sugar is toxic and addictive". Cutting these things out would "cleanse" and "detox" you. It was cult-like in a way and it was easy to get swept up in this community that seemed governed by rules and major health claims that were backed up more by trending hashtags than actual science.

'I would go to these cafes in London's Notting Hill and order £10 smoothies that had moss in them. Why the f*** would I want to drink moss? They were absolutely disgusting, but we all pretended we loved them as we posted enthusiastically on our Instagram accounts with our thousands of followers that were growing by the day.'

Ellie: What was your diet like back then?

Pixie: 'At the start, I stopped eating meat and fish. Then I cut out dairy, eggs, gluten and sugar. In fact, if you followed all those Instagram wellness diets to the letter, you wouldn't even be able to drink water because that's bad for us now too apparently. That's how crazy it's become. And then there were the quite sinister and potentially harmful claims about certain foods curing cancer or depression. This idea that you're somehow to blame if you become ill but that the power to cure yourself lies in cutting out sugar and drinking £10 smoothies is so wrong because health is far more complex than this.

'But it's very easy to fall for a lot of the health claims that are bandied around on social media and online. I was vulnerable to it myself because I was young and anxious about a recent health scare. Other people come to it from a place of being recently diagnosed with an illness or because they have deep-seated issues with food, or perfectionist tendencies or anxiety around food. Some people have unresolved childhood trauma around food – either they were deprived of it by their parents or caregivers so now seek it out in abundance to feel loved. Or they were given certain foods as a source of comfort when they were sad, so are over-reliant on them in adulthood as an emotional comfort blanket, rather than seeing food as something simply to nourish and fuel them.

'Some people are lonely and enjoy being swept up in a community, which from the outside seems so kind and welcoming. I do think a lot of the wellness advice out there is well meaning. It is just very misinformed.'

Ellie: What changed for you?

Pixie: 'Gradually I began to grow weary of the wellness world. I became annoyed by all these bloggers who were pretending to be experts when they were unqualified, and I began writing posts telling my followers not to listen to unqualified experts. But obviously I was also unqualified, so I completed a master's degree in nutrition so that I wouldn't be a hypocrite and it was one of the best decisions I ever made. It's why I'm so passionate now about science-backed health advice, because I know what it's like to fall for misinformation.'

Ellie: What do you think about healthy eating now?

Pixie: 'I now believe there is no such thing as a "bad" food, many of which have become so demonised in recent years. It's all about context. Take alcohol, for example. If you drink wine every night because you're stressed, lonely, bored or anxious, then pretty soon you're going to feel terrible. But that doesn't mean alcohol is "bad" and must be cut out. A nice, cold glass of good wine with a friend over a midweek dinner or a bottle of your favourite red shared with your family over a Sunday roast will leave you feeling nourished and relaxed. There is no good or bad food. Food is context dependent.

'That raw vegan birthday cake may have ticked a lot of health boxes, but it left me feeling flat. Now that I have a healthy, balanced and nourishing diet, I know a slice of gooey chocolate fudge cake won't do me any harm at all. Food is there to be enjoyed after all. For thousands of years food has been used to celebrate weddings, birthdays and festivals and mark important dates in religious calendars. It unites families around dinner tables, and often forms the basis of first or second dates. Having coffee or lunch with a good friend can lift us out of a fog and help us feel comforted and understood. Food has the very real power to connect us to loved ones and tie families together.

'And we know from research that one of the biggest factors in longevity is spending time with other humans. One of the few things that every person on this planet has in common is that they eat – and that's a wonderful thing!'

Ellie: What sort of problems do you help people with now?

> *Pixie:* 'I now have my own private nutrition counselling practice where I see a lot of clients who are confused about what is healthy for them. When they first come to see me they often have a long list of what they perceive as "good" or "bad" foods and conflicting rules about what they should and shouldn't eat. For example, a flapjack made from oats and raisins from a supermarket is "bad", but an organic granola bar made with goji berries or some obscure ingredient is seen as healthy. What makes one food "better" or morally superior to others? The only major difference between them is often the price tag.'

Ellie: What do you think of so-called 'clean eating'?

> *Pixie:* 'I find the language around it moralistic and overly simplistic. I don't agree with attaching a moral value to food, because if certain foods that meet a set of criteria are "clean" that automatically makes those that don't meet the criteria "dirty". And I don't agree with that. Food doesn't have the power to make you a good or bad person. That's giving it far too much power. As my birthday cake showed, it's context dependent. We need to broaden our idea of what healthy means.
>
> 'So much focus is put on how food affects our physical health – its calorie content, how much fat or carbohydrate it contains, its vitamins and minerals. And that stuff is important and has a place. But its benefit on our social and mental health also needs to be taken into consideration. Within the context of a healthy, balanced diet, a pizza and wine night with your friends who really, really make you laugh is prioritising your social and mental health, which needs just as much focus as your physical health.
>
> 'Food can do so much for you – it can help improve your mood, your concentration and your energy levels. It can strengthen your bonds with friends, family and loved ones. And if made well, it tastes amazing, too. So however you eat, I would advise you to do it with as much joy as possible.'

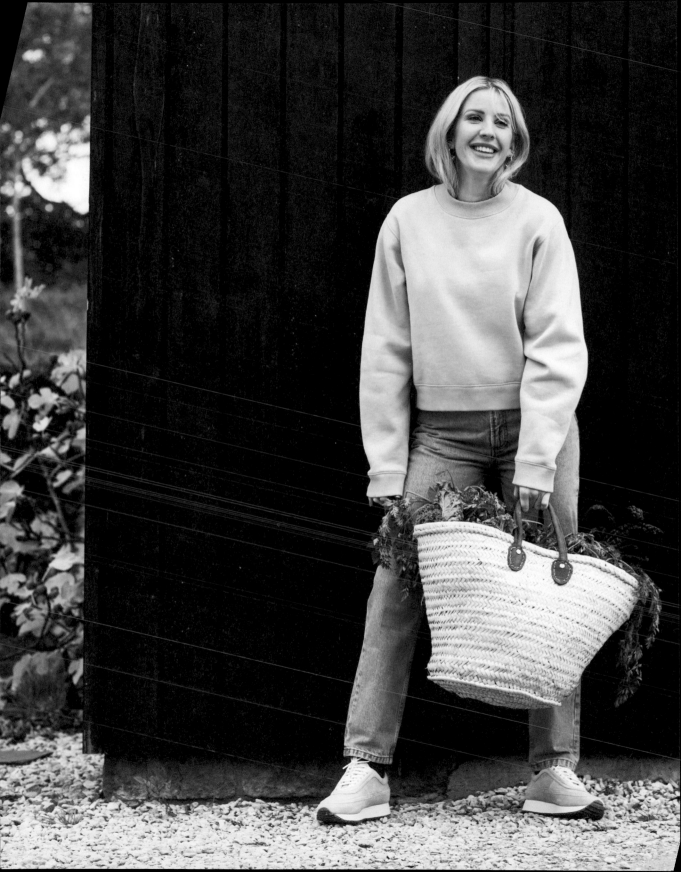

A few food principles (I try to stick to) . . .

I love Pixie's approach and it has really informed my approach to food: overall I keep things really flexible, but I try and bear these principles in mind.

1.   Listen to your body. We underestimate it so much. If we are deficient in something it will make it pretty obvious.

2.   Connect more with what you eat. I think of this as mindful eating. Instead of shopping randomly in the supermarket without knowing the origins of products, I question the impact of things like animal welfare and intensive farming on the planet. I get a real buzz out of supporting local producers and food stores. When I know the backstory or provenance of ingredients, I feel more connected and more relaxed and that makes me really enjoy cooking produce that is from an ethical supply chain.

3.   I try to cook and eat with purpose. Now obviously the purpose of cooking should be to eat it, but as obvious as this sounds it must need reiterating because one-third of all food that we buy ends up in the bin. Can you believe that? The environmental impact of this waste is catastrophic. I've become really passionate about supporting schemes and people who are trying to stop food waste. Some of it is driven by insane standards (we're back to perfection again). Retailers often demand that farmers grade carrots and other veg and fruit on cosmetic grounds. This means 'ugly' veg gets binned. Oddbox.co.uk is an example of a veg box delivery that saves ugly produce and gets it to us (it still tastes good!). The Olioex app allows you to share food in your neighbourhood. So if you do end up with extra – no need to panic!

4.   Fast food doesn't have to mean junk food. Sometimes I have less than 10 minutes to cook, so I chuck a bunch of vegetables and tofu in a pan with some coconut oil and garlic, add a few herbs, and then some cauliflower rice, and I feel like, even though rushed, I've managed to get a good meal in – and it tastes great, too.

5.   Drink lots and lots of water. You cannot underestimate the importance of staying hydrated.

6.   Become a meat-reducer. We don't need to eat meat every day – whatever you were told as a kid – so see if you can shift out of the habit. One of the huge benefits is that you might find yourself trying new foods and flavours that you've never had before. So many of my friends have switched to diets that are predominantly plant-based (obviously I shifted when I was a teenager). My friends who've done this, and now eat meat very sporadically, point out that this is a more cost-effective way to shop and eat, too. Those who do eat meat occasionally buy for quality and knowledge – so they prioritise organic or free-range produce.

7.   Cut down on dairy as well. I personally don't eat a lot of either dairy or meat. I don't believe either to be particularly good for you in large amounts, and there are links between dairy and IBS and poor gut health (see pages 110–113). Again, I believe they should be mostly saved for celebrations, as they are in so many cultures. As well as good plant-based alternatives to meat, there is now ever-improving plant-based dairy, too.

8.   Eat more fruit, vegetables and nuts – variety is key here, especially if you're vegan or vegetarian. The NHS advises that you eat a minimum of five portions of fruit and vegetables a day, but I aim for at least eight portions and at least one of these will be leafy green veggies. My freezer is always full of frozen fruit as well, which are great for smoothies (see recipes in Chapter 8).

9.   Be a smart vegan. Being vegan is so brilliant for your body – and for the planet – but only if you plan properly and make sure you still get all the nutrients you need every day. You need to be a smart vegan to stay in optimum health. See Pixie Turner's advice on this on page 105.

10.   Eat more good fats – not all fats are equal. Good fats come from all sorts of places (avocado, nuts, eggs) and the list of benefits is endless …

11.   Get out of your comfort zone and try new foods – I hope my recipes included later in the book might provide some inspiration for this.

The importance of staying hydrated

It's easy to drink too little water or too many sugary or caffeinated drinks, but what we drink is key to a healthy, nourishing diet. The NHS website states adults should aim for six to eight glasses of fluid a day, but you'll need slightly more on hot days or when you're exercising.

I've always drunk a lot of water because I know it protects my voice, but staying hydrated also makes the rest of our bodies work better. It flushes out toxins, keeps our digestive system working well, keeps our joints and muscles supple and strong, and it's great for our skin. Every night I go to bed with a bottle of water on my nightstand; I have a few sips before I go to sleep and then take a few gulps when I wake up. Our bodies do a pretty good job of keeping us hydrated while we sleep (it's all part of our cleverly designed circadian rhythm, which is our internal body clock), so if you wake up feeling thirsty or dehydrated – and it's not because you've been drinking the night before – then you're probably not drinking enough water during the day.

I put electrolytes in my water: you can buy them in powdered form in health-food shops and there are some great companies making high-quality electrolytes more accessible for people to take on the go. They're very good at keeping you hydrated. I also drink a lot of tea: builders', green, Earl Grey; I love them all and I take my reusable cup with me everywhere for top-ups of my favourite Pukka teas, which I drink all day.

I also love bulletproof coffee. It was first made available by Dave Asprey, an American who discovered it at a retreat in Tibet and founded the Bulletproof Coffee company. It's really popular in the US and available in the UK at certain health-food stores. I make my own version by putting a spoonful of coconut oil or a little grass-fed butter into your coffee. It's delicious and energising and I find it really sets me up for the day. I stopped these for a bit recently because I felt I was overdoing it on the caffeine, but when I'm feeling a bit more balanced and I've had a long week at work, one of these really hits the spot. I also carry MCT oil sachets around with me, which I often add to hot drinks – they go really well with matcha tea. MCT is an essential fatty acid, extracted from foods like coconut oil, and it's been shown to improve your focus and concentration, lower your blood-sugar levels and help maintain energy levels.

My visit to Throne Farm, Herefordshire

I'm a bit obsessed with the connection between our food and the ground it grew in. Perhaps it's a family thing – my brother is a chef and he is always banging on about the importance of eating in season and eco-farming methods. For me, to visit a farm is such a privilege. Throne Farm has the benefit of being near where I grew up. I always feel such a connection to the land and landscape in Hereford, even though I'm not from a farming family. Throne Farm is in a particularly beautiful corner of Herefordshire, nestled near the Welsh Black Mountains. There's been farming here since the 1600s, and now Throne is run as an organic farm by Stephen Ware, whose grandfather James Ware bought the farm in 1943. The ethos is all about sustainability and keeping this land productive for the future. They grow an amazing selection of potatoes, spinach, kale, apples, pears, honey and herbs. I absolutely love visiting.

I arrived one spring morning straight into the fruit orchard where the Wares also grow their herb crops. Later on, in the asparagus field, they passed me an asparagus spear to try, pulled straight from the ground. Oh my god! It couldn't have been fresher and you could taste that.

Organic farming is a system that avoids using pesticides and other agrichemicals. The farmers in an organic system work with the rhythms of the ecosystem, they don't try and beat them using loads of chemicals. Crops are grown in rotation, and the health of the soil is paramount. To see this system in action on such a beautiful farm is a thing of beauty to me. It couldn't be more different from trudging zombie-like around a supermarket buying uniform-perfect produce wrapped in plastic.

How to eat in season

A farm visit or even a trip to a farmers' market (where the ethos is that produce comes from under a 100-mile radius) always boosts my commitment to eat better, for myself and for the planet. One of the ways of doing this is to eat in season.

We've kind of lost touch with this and it's hardly surprising. The average supermarket aisle very much gives the impression that you can have strawberries in December if the mood takes you.

But if you think back, to only a few years ago, you can probably connect with seasonality. When I was growing up, we picked our own strawberries in June and foraged blackberries from local bushes in September.

Wherever possible now, I try to eat seasonal and locally sourced foods, which have been found to be richer in nutrients because they've travelled fewer miles to get to our plates and therefore gone through fewer processes, including different chilling methods, too. Doing this also helps ease us out of 'food ruts' (remember my tour addiction to salad and chips? Well, that was a food rut!) by encouraging us to try a variety of new foods every few months. And they are also kinder to the environment.

Organic food can be more expensive, so I would say buy what you can afford and think about what organic food you decide to buy. For example, you may decide to prioritise organic milk or meat, or perhaps fruit and vegetables. It does frustrate me that there is such a cost difference, and that some mainstream retailers still don't carry very many organic lines. It's such a contrast to other countries like Denmark, where you'll see mainstream supermarkets proudly displaying organic products out front.

WHAT FRUIT AND VEG TO EAT, SEASON BY SEASON . . .

SPRING
(March to May):

Apples

Apricots

Asparagus

Baby carrots

Broccoli

Cauliflower

Purple sprouting broccoli

Rhubarb

Salad leaves

Spinach

Spring onions

SUMMER
(June to August):

Beans

Beetroot

Blueberries

Carrots

Cherries

Courgettes

Fennel

Mangetout

Melon

New potatoes

Peas

Plums

Rocket

Shallots

Spinach

Strawberries

Sweetcorn

Tomatoes

Watercress

AUTUMN
(September to November):

Apples

Aubergines

Beetroot

Blackberries

Broad beans

Brussels sprouts

Cabbage

Cauliflower

Celery

Cranberries

Kale

Leek

Nectarines

Parsnips

Pears

Potatoes

Squash

Wild mushrooms

WINTER
(December to February):

Apples

Broccoli

Brussels sprouts

Cauliflower

Celeriac

Clementine

Figs

Kale

Pumpkin

Shallots

Squash

Swede

Turnip

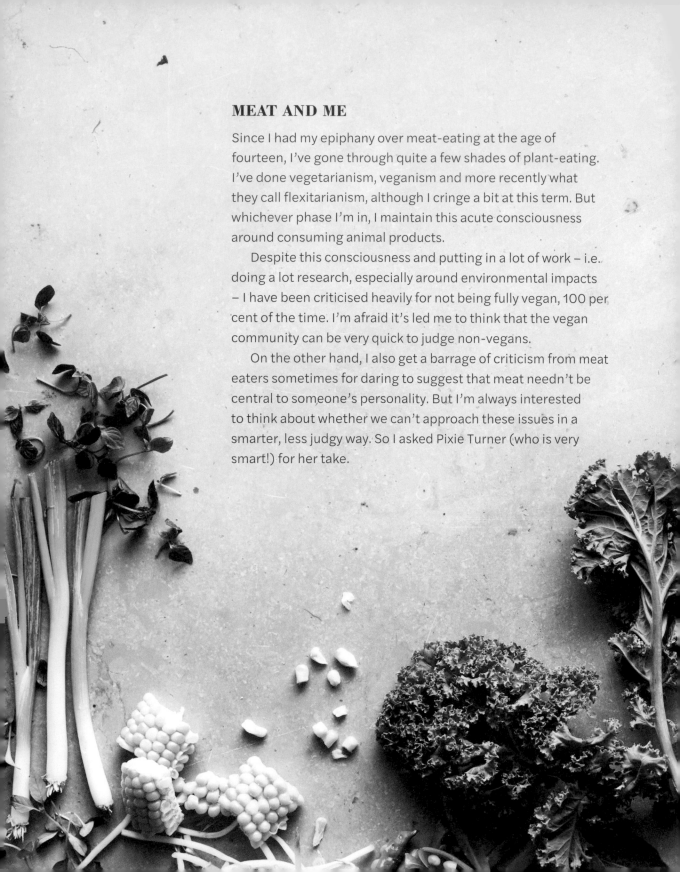

MEAT AND ME

Since I had my epiphany over meat-eating at the age of fourteen, I've gone through quite a few shades of plant-eating. I've done vegetarianism, veganism and more recently what they call flexitarianism, although I cringe a bit at this term. But whichever phase I'm in, I maintain this acute consciousness around consuming animal products.

Despite this consciousness and putting in a lot of work – i.e. doing a lot research, especially around environmental impacts – I have been criticised heavily for not being fully vegan, 100 per cent of the time. I'm afraid it's led me to think that the vegan community can be very quick to judge non-vegans.

On the other hand, I also get a barrage of criticism from meat eaters sometimes for daring to suggest that meat needn't be central to someone's personality. But I'm always interested to think about whether we can't approach these issues in a smarter, less judgy way. So I asked Pixie Turner (who is very smart!) for her take.

HOW TO BE A SMART VEGAN, BY NUTRITIONIST PIXIE TURNER

'Choosing to go vegan for environmental or ethical reasons is a noble pursuit. Unlike what some sensationalist documentaries will tell you, there are no clear-cut, obvious health benefits to going vegan – the healthfulness of your diet depends on what you are eating, not what you're excluding. And if you are planning on going vegan, there are a few nutrition considerations to make.

'First, a vitamin B12 supplement is essential and non-negotiable in my eyes. This vitamin is found pretty exclusively in animal products, and while fortified plant milks can give you a little, I recommend taking a daily supplement to be certain of a regular intake.

'Secondly, an algae-based omega-3 supplement ensures you're getting those wonderful fats that look after your brain. You'll find omega-3 fats in plant foods like chia seeds and flax seeds, but your body has to convert these to the more useful version, and it's not great at that. So I suggest making life easier for your brain by giving it the form of omega-3 in algae (DHA and/or EPA) that it likes best.

'Finally, a variety of foods is key. Aside from the above, focus less on individual foods and nutrients and more on the overall pattern of what you're eating. Vegan meals are not a problem as long as you're also eating plenty of vegetables alongside them.'

A word on fasting

The benefits of intermittent fasting – where you eat or fast within a set time window – are fairly well documented and include a stronger immune system, sustained energy levels and weight loss. Fasting forces your body to dip into its fat reserves to use them as fuel. The traditional way of eating – three meals a day, with several snacks dotted throughout – keeps your insulin levels high, so your body never taps into its fat stores. Fasting can also reduce levels of IGF-1, which is an insulin-like growth factor, that leads to accelerated ageing, plus it can reduce your blood pressure, cholesterol and glucose (blood-sugar) levels.

When you try traditional dieting and take in fewer calories, your body rebels by holding on to what calories you do consume and makes you hungrier.

When you fast, however, even for 5–6 hours, your body starts tapping in to those fat stores as energy, plus it gives your digestion a much-needed break. I've tried fasting a few times. Initially I found the novelty exciting. I would spend the whole day being productive and I realised it was because I wasn't basing my day around mealtimes. I found that when I fasted the first thing I wanted to eat to break the fast was something nutritious, like a huge salad, because my body was craving the good stuff.

Fasting also gives me a lot of mental clarity and that boosted my creative capacity (in a sense, I felt able to work harder for longer and achieve more). Yes, the first few days I did it, I thought a lot about burgers and fries. But by the fourth day, your brain starts to accept that no food will be consumed for a good few hours so it may as well concentrate on something else.

My approach to fasting now is that I employ it for a bit, when I feel like I need it. Sometimes it's as simple as not eating anything after 8 p.m. and until 8 a.m. the next morning (you should always give your digestion a good break overnight – at least eleven or twelve hours). Sometimes I extend it and eat my last meal by 8 p.m. and then I won't eat until midday the following day. That's a sixteen-hour fast and it's surprisingly easy, especially if you're not much of a breakfast person. Fasted workouts, where you exercise on an empty stomach, are good and encourage your body to use fat (rather than carbohydrates) as fuel. However, it's important to stay hydrated and keep to a level of intensity you feel comfortable with. I wouldn't go to Barry's Bootcamp on an empty stomach, for example, because it's such a hard workout.

A word of warning, though: fasting isn't for everybody and it's not recommended if you're pregnant or breastfeeding, have a history of eating disorders or take medication for diabetes. If you are thinking of giving it a try and have any health concerns, make sure you speak to your GP first.

Why you need to stop thinking fat is bad

From the 1980s onwards, low-fat diets reigned supreme and were touted as the best way to stay slim and healthy by doctors, dieticians and the food industry, who were keen to make as many low-fat foods as possible to entice us all to buy into the idea that fat-free was best.

Forty years on, and despite countless studies that show how crucial a role fat plays in our diet, the low-fat ideal still has a hold on many of us. Often without thinking, we pick out processed margarine spreads over pure butter, we order a skinny flat white or choose the low-fat Greek yoghurt, and we buy low-fat cereals or porridges, thinking they're the best way to start the day.

I used to think fat was the devil. Growing up, it was fat-free this and fat-free that. I would eat low-fat yoghurts in my teens, convinced I was being healthy, despite the fact that they were packed full of sugar and artificial sweeteners. I didn't realise then that our bodies can cope perfectly well with natural fat – they can break it down, digest it, put it to good use in boosting our brain power and concentration, getting our digestion to work well, and lubricating and improving mobility in our joints – but don't really have any use for sugar, so it just turns to fat, which our body stubbornly holds on to.

For years, I thought having a low-fat diet was key, which is why I suffered from IBS symptoms, headaches and a lack of energy; all of which I put down to my frenzied schedule. Now I love healthy fats and eat them every day; eggs, avocado, nuts and seeds. Organic meat and cheese are also a good source, although I don't really eat either very often.

Our bodies need fat from food because it's an important source of energy. It helps our bodies absorb important vitamins and minerals, it's essential for our metabolism, it oils our joints and it plumps up our skin. People on fat-free diets – especially those eating a lot of sugar, or artificially sweetened food in the place of fat – will often notice it in their complexion.

Of course, when it comes to fat, some fats are better than others. The best type of dietary fat is found in oily fish, nuts and seeds, avocado, eggs, flax seeds, coconut butter and milk.

The fat found in oily fish – like mackerel and salmon – and nuts, seeds, oils and avocados contains essential fatty acids, which boost overall health, including the formation of healthy cell membranes, brain function, hormone production, the regulation of blood pressure and liver function, improved thyroid activity and healthy skin and hair. The list goes on . . .

The fats found in organic meat or poultry are also beneficial, but don't eat red meat every day. When it comes to meat generally, my advice is to eat it occasionally and buy the best you can.

The fats to avoid include processed, non-organic red meats, like bacon, ham, mince and the like. Now I never question why a cut of meat is so expensive, but rather why a pack of meat is so cheap. I also avoid trans fats, which are a form of processed, hydrogenated cooking oil used to prolong a food's shelf life and add flavour. Trans fats serve no nutritional purpose, but they have been shown to raise our risk of heart disease, certain cancers and obesity. Trans fats can often be found in fast foods like doughnuts, muffins, biscuits and crisps. Not all of these foods contain trans fats – and manufacturers in the UK have largely stopped using them in their foods – but it's always worth checking the ingredients for terms like, 'hydrogenated oil' or 'hydrogenated vegetable oil', which is basically a trans fat.

Lastly, good fat tastes great (actually, bad fats found in shop-bought muffins with a ten-year expiry date can also taste delicious, but a funny kind of delicious and they're terrible for you, so try to avoid them!). Healthy fat adds a natural flavour to our foods, fills us up and stops us from overeating. It's very easy to overeat a large bowl of cereal or pasta, which is comparatively low in fat. Yet half an avocado sprinkled with pumpkin seeds or a couple of poached eggs with a side of smoked salmon will keep you full and nourished for hours. So don't fear fat, just make sure you choose it wisely.

Listen to your gut

Gut health is something that I have really spent a lot of time thinking about, researching and experimenting with lately. I've discovered that our gut health plays such an important role in improving our entire body health and wellbeing, with various studies over the last few years highlighting the strong link between our gut health and our overall health, including our mental health. There are about eleven trillion bacterial cells – known as our microbiome – living all over and inside our body, and the largest concentration is in our gut. Isn't that incredible? One day I want to visit the University of Reading where they've created a version of the human gut in a laboratory to test probiotics and carry out other fascinating research on microbiomes (by the way, they call it the fart lab, which obviously I find hilarious).

Having a wide range of friendly bacteria is best, so eat a wide variety of vegetables and fruit, which feed the good bacteria in your gut. The same food day in and day out isn't great for our guts, or microbiome. These gut bacteria also digest fibre from high-fibre foods, like grains and beans, so fibre is crucial for gut health. A healthy microbiome will also keep our weight nice and steady, because the bacteria in our gut interacts with the hormones in our gut that regulate our appetite, such as leptin and ghrelin. Below, I've listed a few ways to keep your gut in good shape.

But what can leave our microbiome depleted? As well as inflaming our guts, too much alcohol can cause unfriendly bacteria to overtake friendly bacteria. Sensible drinking is OK, but too much or too frequent drinking isn't great for your microbiome. Similarly, too much sugar, artificially sweetened foods and caffeine can be quite tough on your gut, so keep an eye on your intake and listen to how your body reacts to them.

Ways to improve your gut health

KEEP A FOOD DIARY

This goes back to my sugary cereal and cornflake-and-milk days. Every time I ate a bowl, within a few minutes my stomach would start to whirl and contract, which would lead to bloating and uncomfortable digestive symptoms. You may find your gut triggers are cows' milk, too much wine, one too many coffees, cheese, or rich, fatty foods. That doesn't mean you have to cut these foods out, but it does mean you should keep an eye on how your body – and crucially your gut – reacts to them. Your gut is your very own nutritionist, so listen to it carefully.

KEEP AN EYE ON YOUR STRESS

Ever wondered why you get 'butterflies' in the pit of your stomach before a job interview or first date? Or why you can't eat when you're scared? We literally feel our emotions in our gut because of the link between our gut and our brain. Our gut is full of nerves, so when we feel stressed, scared, anxious or fearful, our body diverts its energy away from the digestive system and instead turns its attention to our muscles and pumps out the stress hormones cortisol and adrenaline. This is an evolutionary throwback to the days when we literally needed to flee a predator. Which was great news in the past if you needed to run away from a tiger prowling around your cave or an arrow heading your way. But terrible news for your poor gut if you're weighed down with day-to-day stress like deadlines, too much social media, a bad relationship or demanding boss. Over time, chronic stress can take a toll on your digestive system and lead to bloating, indigestion, stomach cramps or loss of appetite (which can then cause you to binge later on because you haven't eaten properly or regularly enough).

Lastly, don't eat when you're stressed, working or on a deadline, because your gut will be so busy focusing on the stress of what you're doing, it won't do its job of digesting your food properly. Wait, let the stress pass or finish your work, and then eat in a calm and screen-free way.

EAT REGULARLY

Just like a regular sleeping pattern (going to bed and waking up at the same time) helps the quality of your sleep, eating your meals at roughly the same time each day keeps your digestive system ticking over nicely. Start each day with a glass of warm water and lemon and sip it slowly. Try not to drink too much coffee before breakfast because this can sometimes trigger a reaction in your gut, and don't gulp down drinks with your meals because this can also unsettle an overloaded digestive system.

EAT FIBRE

Fibre is good for 'moving things along', but do be careful not to eat too much, as this can be hard to digest and can make IBS symptoms worse. Soaking oats in milk (either cows' milk or a non-dairy alternative) can make them easier to digest, and cooked fruits and vegetables are also easier to digest than raw ones. And again, don't forget to drink plenty of water. Sipping it slowly, little and often, will help to grease the wheels of your digestive system.

TRY FERMENTED FOODS

Fermented foods like kimchi, sauerkraut and sourdough bread, and drinks like kefir and kombucha, have all been found to improve the health of your digestion by increasing the 'good' bacteria in your gut. You can make your own (see recipe on page 256) or buy them easily from most good supermarkets.

Rather than rushing out and bulk-buying all of the ones mentioned here, start slowly and see how your gut feels after adding small amounts of one or two of these to your meals or morning routine.

EAT A VARIED DIET

Finally, as Pixie tells us, our gut loves a wide variety of different foods. It's not good for our gut to eat the same things day in and day out – again I can only apologise to my gut for the years of salad 'n' chips. This is just one reason why it's so important to experiment in the kitchen and try out some new food combinations. It's also a joyous thing to do. So I hope my recipes in Chapter 8 might provide some new ideas.

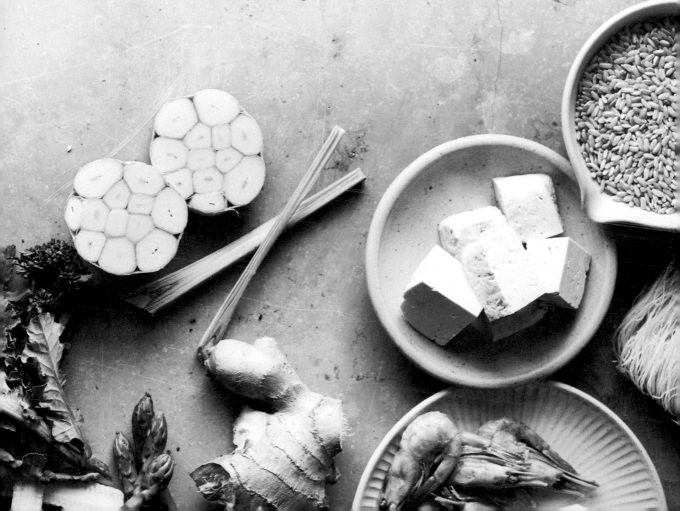

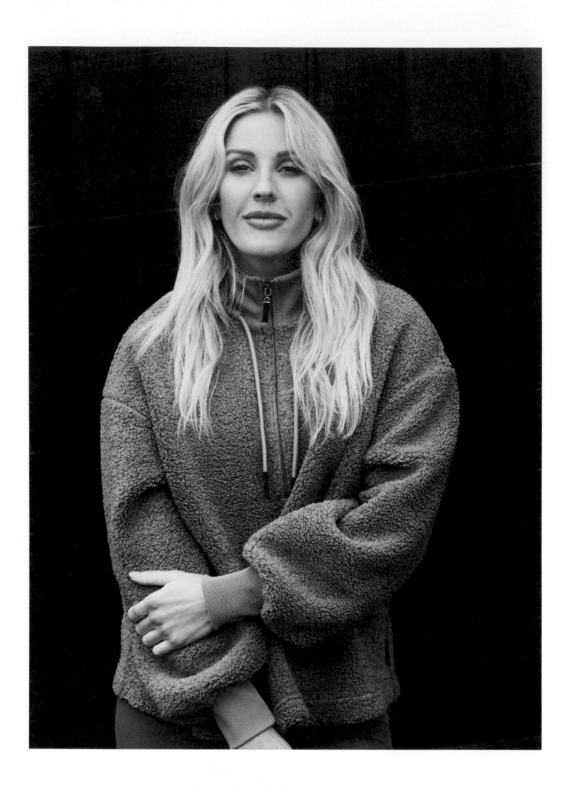

5

THE MINDSET RESET

'Your strongest muscle is your mind.
Train it well.'

ANON

Half the effort involved in starting or doing a workout comes from your mind. I've heard people say that their minds carried them through the second half of a marathon just as much as, if not more than, their feet and muscles. Everything begins with your mindset. If you're not familiar with thinking about mindsets, it's very simple. Your mindset is a collection of your opinions and beliefs that influences your behaviour. If your collection is all about how rubbish everything is, you will find it hard to come up with dynamic, constructive patterns of behaviour. If your mindset is open and positive, that sort of change will be much easier. As you don't inherit this collection, you can decide to swap them for different ones. Change your mindset and a change in your actions will follow.

Nike created the best marketing slogan of all time when they came up with 'Just Do It'. That's what we should all tell ourselves about exercise. If you're new to exercise, the first few times you do it will be tough. There is no point making excuses, and yet we all do it. I continue to do it. Excuses I have tried to make (to myself by the way) to excuse myself from running include 'wrong sort of grip on shoes. I might slip', 'fake tan might run due to sweat' (not so much now, but in the 2000s) and 'can't find hair bobble'. It's as if I am thirteen and trying to get out of PE. But never mind. The excuses are weak, and deep down I know that. These days, after I've wasted a few minutes pretending I'm not going to go, I . . . go for a run and, guess what, then I feel happy and energised. I don't always want to work out, but once I've done it I never, ever regret it. Nobody ever regrets a workout. (And we can't say that often enough, so I'll keep saying it in this book and beyond!)

I find it helps to think of my body as a machine – an amazing machine that's more than capable of anything I set out to do with it. It may take a little time to warm up, or to get fitter or faster, but in time, and with practice, you will realise your body is so much stronger than you think it is. You'll also realise your body is designed to move. Whether that's running, stretching, lifting or bending, our bodies were created with movement in mind. Evolutionarily, we are designed to be able to walk for miles looking for food, and to run away from sabre-toothed tigers and other dangers; we evolved to survive, and that meant moving.

If you think of your body as a capable, strong machine that thrives on movement, it will motivate you to move it every day.

Our body is the greatest gift we'll ever have, so the least we can do is feed it well and keep up a good level of fitness. Whenever I'm looking for motivation to exercise, I just think about how we've all been given these incredible bodies and how great it feels when we look after them properly. I feel so grateful to have a healthy, working body with blood pumping around it that delivers oxygen and nutrients to my muscles, which are strong and able.

Or sometimes, when I'm struggling to stay motivated, I think about how crap I feel when I don't exercise or when I eat junk food night after night. I think about how sluggish and tired those things make me feel. For me, that is motivation enough. It's hard to find any more excuses when I remember that.

'It always seems impossible until it is done'

NELSON MANDELA , FORMER PRESIDENT OF SOUTH AFRICA

Athleticism over aesthetics

You also need to remember why you're eating well or exercising. For me, it's about being a strong and physically powerful woman. It's about feeling uplifted and capable. It's about being energised and feeling alive. I want to be athletic and fit and the very best version of myself that I can be. I won't lie, a happy by-product of living well is having a flatter stomach and toned thighs – I like the way my body looks when I'm healthy – but how I feel is far more important to me. Feeling strong and energised is the most motivating sensation you can have, much more powerful than having the perfect face or perfect body. I'm not saying don't enjoy and appreciate those things, but they shouldn't be your motivation for training or eating a certain way. Do it to feel better, not to look better – then you will enjoy the journey as much as the result. And make sure you're doing it for you.

It's so liberating and empowering being physically strong as a woman. It changes the way you walk, the way you smile; it changes your confidence, and how you look at others and exchange with them. It changes everything about your being. I sometimes get social anxiety when I walk into a room and everybody looks at me. I get it in other situations, too, often for no obvious reason. But when I work out, it gives me an underlying confidence that helps with my social anxiety. It feels like I have a new tool in my armoury. I'm ready for whatever life throws at me. That feeling goes far beyond thinking you look OK in clothes.

'Set your goals high enough to inspire you, and low enough to encourage you'

ANON

Now is the time to start questioning the limitations you put on yourself: 'I don't have time. I'm not strong enough. I'm not a naturally athletic person. I don't enjoy running. I don't feel like working out is my thing.' Are those things really true or are they just things you tell yourself?

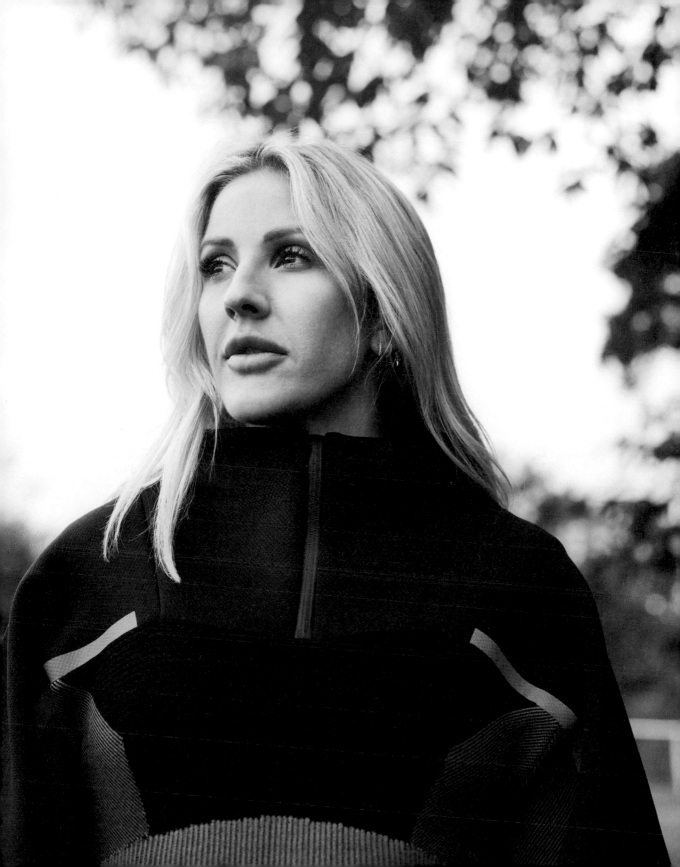

Meet . . . DR TAMSIN LEWIS

Dr Tamsin is a medical doctor who qualified with honours from King's College London and Guys and St Thomas' Hospital. She works in lifestyle and preventative medicine.

As well as a BSc in neuroscience and the biology of ageing, Dr Tamsin has specialist training in psychiatry and is a member of the Royal College of Psychiatrists. She is interested in our behaviour around health, which I find fascinating. She has also trained in sports medicine, with further education in nutritional and functional medicine and is a former GB elite triathlete and an Ironman champion.

I was first introduced to her in 2018 by my then boxing coach, Shane, son of the legendary boxer Barry McGuigan. Tamsin is a huge inspiration to me and a great friend. I had a really interesting chat with her about mindset and learned behaviours.

Ellie: We've been working together for a few years now. In that time you have taught me so much about mindset. What is it about human mindset and behaviour that you find so interesting?

Dr Tamsin: 'I became fascinated by the concept of human potential as part of my own journey through childhood adversity, a traumatic brain injury and depression, to winning an Ironman triathlon at my first attempt when I was (unknowingly) pregnant.

'That day, laying over the finish line, head in hands in tears, I shook my head to myself in disbelief. I had not thought I could complete the distance of a 2.4-mile swim, a 112-mile bike ride and a marathon (26.2 miles). I had never even run a marathon before, let alone preceded one with a bike ride and run. It was my coach who believed I could, and together we worked on the "possibility mindset".'

Ellie: What is that?

Dr Tamsin: 'Possibility mindset is an approach to training. It is based around the theory that you become what you repeatedly do and believe you can do. Possibility mindset is different from positive mindset or positive thinking. Possibility mindset helps you look at the future and make the switch from thinking something is impossible to believing it's possible. It's about breaking goals or problems down into bite-size chunks and seeing the possibility for change within them. Over time, relying on small, incremental changes to your routine – where you put yourself through slight discomfort – you nudge your body and brain to evolve.

'With possibility mindset you reflect on what you did differently. You think about how it felt, you praise yourself and accept the praise of others for your progress, however small it is. It helps to track trends, and this is where the learnings from my time as a professional athlete affected my practice as a medical doctor. This concept of a "possibility mindset" drives human potential.'

Ellie: So this comes back to the idea that we're capable of more than we realise?

Dr Tamsin: 'Yes, exactly. We have all heard the notion of "mind over matter", and that we are capable of far more than we think we are. I'm interested in how we actually take steps to realise this potential.

'I came at this originally through a medical lens and then I focused on it more during my time as an athlete. The concept of marginal gains (see page 123) is magnified in the context of sporting excellence. I learned that by measuring and modifying your physical health you could change your mental health and mindset, which then determines how you interact with your environment day to day.'

Ellie: How do you mean?

> *Dr Tamsin:* 'Anyone who has been anaemic can tell you that the low energy that results from it makes you draw inwards, reduce activities that tire you and effectively over time change what your life looks like.
>
> 'The same goes for hormones, women change their activities and mood and food choices throughout the month without thinking about it as their hormone levels fluctuate over the course of their menstrual cycle. The high testosterone peak in the middle of the month sees you more assertive, with a higher libido, and is the ideal time to reap the rewards from any strength work.
>
> 'There are many more examples, but the point is your biochemistry determines how you interact with the world – and vice versa. We are dynamic beings, constantly in flux with our environment. The "possibility mindset" allows us to begin to see this and make choices that help us to grow. It takes commitment, but with small nudges towards a new sense of self, all the while knowing it is OK to fall backwards or simply fall and get back up, I have seen many people flourish with this approach.'

Ellie: You have often talked to me about the importance of resilience as well. Can you tell me what resilience means to you?

> *Dr Tamsin:* 'Resilience is strength within, but it relies on the ability to draw upon internal and external resources. Internal resources are things like optimism, mindfulness, savouring positive memories and breathwork. External resources include support groups, therapists, doctors, friends, yoga and exercise classes, nutritionists, and so on. Then there are physical tools you can use as well. These include things like cold-water immersion, which can also help to build resilience.'

Ellie: What are 'marginal gains'?

Dr Tamsin: 'Marginal gains are a series of small changes and incremental improvements that result in a big difference to results and outcome. There are different ways of applying marginal gains, but some elite athletes think of it in terms of small, daily improvements of 1 per cent in all areas of whatever type of training they are doing. For instance, Ellie, I know you love your running. So you'd look at every element of that – your breathing, increase effectiveness by 1 per cent; your race tactics, increase by 1 per cent; and so on. There's fitness and conditioning, of course, but there are other things that might seem on the periphery, like sleeping in the right position, having the same pillow when you are away . . . they're tiny things but if you clump them together it makes a big difference.'

I find talking to Dr Tam raises my ambition levels when it comes to my own training, and I particularly love this 1-per-cent method and find it so refreshing as an outlook. And it can be used in any area of your life – your fitness goals, your diet, your business or your relationships.

It all relies on the theory that making small changes – tiny tweaks to improve things, day in and day out – can lead to better results than one big change. Anyone who has ever gone on a January diet or juice fast will know this. When you make those big, sweeping, life-altering changes, full of rigid routines, they can feel completely overwhelming and unsustainable, so more often than not we quit them. But if we increase our accomplishments by just 1 per cent – for me, that might mean going that little bit further on a run; adding in a little hill; running a little faster or for a little longer; piling my plate slightly higher with greens; eating a little less chocolate (particularly hard for me); spending a little less time on my phone; going to bed a bit earlier – big improvements can start to happen.

Most importantly, changing our habits by such a small amount feels doable. Unlike a strict January diet that ends in failure (and a sweeties binge) in February, making small changes that quietly and easily become habits makes us feel capable and proud. And this strengthens our mindset and keeps us wanting to make more changes, because we know we can stick to them and that they make a difference to how we feel.

The power of goal setting

While I don't agree with wearable or fitness trackers dictating our every move, I do think they can play an important role in goal setting and motivation. I have experimented with so many over time – the Oura Ring, the WHOOP band, the Polar Vantage, the Fitbit – but you may also find one of the many other trackers and health and fitness tracking apps helpful.*

One of the most useful things for me is how they remind you to move a bit more. Sometimes I'll be busy pottering about – cooking, food shopping, walking, cleaning the house – and I'll realise I've done a lot more activity than I thought. Other times I'll realise I've barely moved all day, and the tracker is a good reminder to get up and move. Maybe I'll do a few squats while I'm brushing my teeth (balancing on one leg is good for brain training, too!) or march on the spot when I'm washing up.

Some people think movement doesn't count if it doesn't take place in the gym, but your body will thank you for any movement – it just wants you to move. My trainer Matt, who you'll hear from in the following chapter, says that people will often do an hour's workout in the gym and then tick a box in their head that tells them they've done their movement for the day, so they can relax on the sofa. The result is that they don't

* We also discuss this in Chapter 2, 'Listen to Your Body'.

keep their fitness levels up but can't work out why. It's fine to relax on the sofa, by the way, but the point Matt's making is that, even if you go to the gym, you should still move the rest of the time. I might lie on the sofa in the evening watching TV, but every 15–20 minutes I make a conscious effort to get up and stretch or squat, or just move my body, going from one room to the next, or find an excuse to jog up the stairs to get something.

Becoming conscious of your body's need for movement is similar to me to forming an environmental conscience. I have campaigned on behalf of the planet for many years (I became a global ambassador for the UN Environment Programme in 2017) so I know that once you become aware of the Nature and Climate Crisis you are always aware. It means you become mindful of everything around you and everything you do.

That includes stuff like being super-aware of what you consume – including buying too many 'fast-fashion' clothes that have a heavy environmental impact. And becoming really cross when items are delivered in swathes of plastic packaging (plastic will be with us for hundreds of years, and each year eight million tonnes goes into our oceans). The point is when you know stuff like this, you can't forget it. Everything you do becomes geared to being more sustainable. It's the same with movement. Once you become aware of how important movement is, you'll become mindful of moving your body every day and you'll begin to thrive on it.

'It doesn't matter how slowly you go, so long as you don't stop'

CONFUCIUS, CHINESE PHILOSOPHER AND POLITICIAN

My mindset rules

Remember you are supposed to be fit and healthy and function well. This is your default (or factory setting), not feeling crappy. In order to reach your body and mind's full potential, emotionally and physically, you need to give your body and mind what it needs!

Get to the point where you are your own motivation and you don't need anybody else to encourage you to go out on a run or to a gym class. Do it for you and you alone.

Throw out any old, negative habits that are keeping you in a rut. Make new ones – you don't have to save New Year's Resolutions for the start of a year. Just call them 'Resolutions' instead!

You DO have time. Stop telling yourself that you don't. Even if you run for 10 minutes, that's 10 minutes more than no run at all. You DO NOT need an hour to exercise. Even 10 minutes is good, to get moving.

Being uncomfortable makes you stronger. Try a longer run than usual, or a new gym class or online trainer. Go for a wild swim or have a cold shower. Raise your tolerance and push yourself out of your comfort zone every once in a while.

Spend some time making a workout playlist – music has been shown to motivate people to exercise for longer and harder.

In the same way you are what you eat, you become what you think. So be mindful of what you focus your attention on.

Think about your mind as well as your body. Remember that exercise and eating well don't just affect your physical body, but your mind, too. They affect the way you think, the way you make decisions and the way you respond to situations.

Feed your mind as well as you feed your body. Seek out positive people. Don't watch too much TV; watch films and documentaries that stir and rouse you instead. Come up with new ideas and be creative. Be selective about who you follow on social media. And don't 'consume' emotional junk. Remember you are the gatekeeper to your mind.

Stop overcomplicating things. You don't need £100 trainers and designer leggings with bum-sculpting technology to exercise. Fitness trackers can be really helpful, but you don't need one. Stop using those things to put off your run by another day. Just get out of your seat and get moving. Even if you move slowly and for not very long – just get up and move! Once you're out of the door and doing a workout, resistance fades.

And finally, remember, nobody has ever regretted a workout.

Tailor your workout to your mood – and know when to give yourself a break

A few months ago I woke up with PMS and I was feeling out of sorts and I decided to jot down how I felt and what I did (or didn't do). I ate a huge amount of chocolate and spent longer lying on the sofa watching TV than I normally would. I knew that was what my body needed. However, I also knew that was just a day – not a habit – and the next day I felt more energised, so I went for a four-mile jog and made a green smoothie when I got home (nice and balanced so as not to cause a spike in glucose!).

This sounds unremarkable, but it's an example of taking a small break in training and routine, dictated by my body, and then quite naturally picking up training afterwards.

My husband Caspar is the opposite: he has an athlete's mindset and is much less emotional about his workouts. He'll wake up and, regardless of how he feels, just go and exercise. And that works for him. Everybody is different. But I'm led by my mood and how my body feels.

The first time you go for a run you may find it scary, but then you'll begin to understand that your body is there to help you run, not work against you. Or maybe running isn't your thing. There are no right or wrong exercises, there's no hierarchy. Just choose the thing you enjoy and go for it.

I try to dress for my morning workouts. When I wake up, the first thing I put on is activewear because it means I'm more likely to move around that day. (That's also the reason I hardly ever wear jeans!)

I also try to match my workout to my mood. If I'm stressed or anxious, a run really helps me. Some people meditate, but I prefer a run; it helps me process my thoughts and also allows me to work off my pent-up energy and stress. Boxing is my go-to when I want to get energised. I love the surge of power and adrenaline that it brings. I never feel stronger (physically or mentally) than after I've just completed my boxing training. The only thing that comes close is being on stage. I love being in cold water as well. Even though it can feel so unpleasant to begin with, you feel amazing afterwards. I try to go cold-water swimming if I need a boost to start my day or I've been feeling a bit low recently.

Yoga is also very important to me. It's always been a constant exercise and while I may not do it every week or even every month, I always come back to it – especially when my mood is all over the place. It's a good balancer. Yoga is so important as you get older because you become less agile with age, and even less agile if you don't stretch your body regularly. Our culture now means we spend so much time sitting in front of a computer or a phone or a TV. But our bodies aren't designed to sit for long periods in the same position, so it's important to counter all that sitting with regular stretching. Yoga really opens up your chest and heart, it gets your digestion moving and also helps you become better at other workouts, like running.

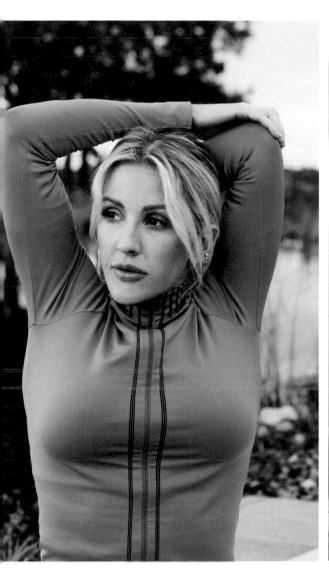
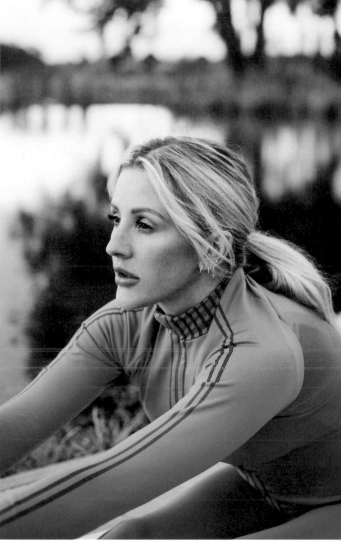

Fill your mind with positive thoughts

Trust me, I know how hard this is. Something happens to me when I first wake up. It is like my brain has only woken up the irrational part – and all I can think about is doom and gloom and that everything is shit. And the part that knows that this is just my old habit of negative thinking coming back to haunt me, and that actually I'm alive, I'm healthy and everything is fine, is still fast asleep. There must be some kind of biological explanation for this!

As you will have seen throughout this book, I am often self-deprecating, and I suppose I have used it as a survival technique for years. If ever I didn't win something, or wasn't invited to something, or just generally felt inadequate, I would put myself down before anyone else could. The people around me would find it funny, so I kept doing it. And then I realised it had become part of my personality and I started to really believe what I was saying and thinking about myself.

So instead I started saying to myself 'I'll win another time', 'I'll perform better next time' or 'I am actually worthy of that, but it wasn't right for me at this time.' And those things then really did start to come true.

So even if you don't believe it, say it. Say that you can do it. And with exercise, keep telling yourself that you can do exactly what you want to achieve, whether it's a 4km run, or lifting heavier weights, or just getting through a HIIT session without dying. Yes, it requires some work and dedication, but it is never impossible, and you should always remind yourself kindly that you'll get there. Remind yourself that you can do it. And remember that the human body is so much more resilient and brilliant than you know – with time, it will do exactly what you want it to.

Read more books

We have got into the habit of constantly checking social media to see what other people are doing, what other people are wearing, how other people are being productive, while completely abandoning ourselves in the process.

In the same way that we read gossip magazines to let our minds drift, we often use social media as a distraction from the things we need to be working on. Very little that is productive ever comes out of social media. So my advice is to stay off social media as much as possible – I promise you that the same shit will be on your timeline in three weeks' time when you eventually go back to it – and spend your time reading some books instead.

The concentration that goes into reading, no matter how easy a read, helps your memory and expands your vocabulary – for all those times when you just can't find the word for what you're trying to explain. It also improves your empathy, because you are taking yourself into other worlds and experiencing and investing in the plight of others. It is even proven to decrease your chances of developing Alzheimer's later in life. Every time I read a book, whether fiction or non-fiction, I feel like I learn something new, and I also learn more about myself through the book.

I love fiction for allowing me to enter new worlds or travel back to the past for romance or sentimentalism and I love non-fiction for the powerful feeling of new understanding it brings.

There are so many books in the world. It overwhelms me to know I will only read the teeniest fraction of them in my lifetime. I believe reading anything at all helps. Pick up the book you've been meaning to read and make yourself read it for at least 20 minutes. I promise you that you'll feel as if you've accomplishedsomething – and you probably won't want to put it down either!

SOME OF MY FAVOURITE BOOKS:

Just Kids by Patti Smith

This book started my lifelong love affair with Patti Smith, just as it documents the beginning of her lifelong affair with art and music. I loved everything about it, especially reading about the excitement and disarray of 1970s New York.

What I Talk About When I Talk About Running by Haruki Murakami

This beautiful memoir is by a Japanese writer who started running in the 1980s and since then has run over twenty marathons and an ultra-marathon. I had never read anything like this before – Murakami's writing is so powerful, he immediately takes you into the unreal, linking his obsessions and exploring themes of sex, loneliness and death. OK, so that's a whole other conversation, but his writing made me realise that having a passion for running is linked to creativity and the way this can heighten your senses.

21 Lessons for the 21st Century by Yuval Noah Harari

Sometimes, as much as you want to watch Love Island or the comforting film you love for the thousandth time, you have to muster everything in you to read a book that confronts the reality of what lies ahead in your own and your children's future. Knowledge is power, and clarity, in a world of fake news, is essential. This book of short essays gives you plenty to think about. From the rise of AI, Trumpism and climate change, to terrorism and religion, it is hard for me to think of a better book to really enlighten yourself on the goings on in the world, and possible reasons for why things have gone a bit wrong. This book also helped me understand addiction to social media.

Human Traces by Sebastian Faulks

I can absolutely recommend every single Sebastian Faulks book, but this is one of my favourites. I love the way he writes with such a beautiful blend of the poetic and the factual. I love his imagery and the way he describes his feelings. This book is about the beginnings of understanding psychology and how the mind works, and is just a really, really great read.

Trick Mirror by Jia Tolentino

There is a lot to take in with this book: themes of social-media addiction; celebrity obsession; our dependence on the internet; and how feminism has been successful but that there are still so many things to overcome and fundamentally change in our social, political and economic systems. Nevertheless, I was gripped from the first page. I highly recommend it.

A New Earth by Eckhart Tolle

This was a follow-up book to his debut, *The Power of Now*. Even if you aren't a particularly spiritual person (I definitely didn't consider myself to be) this book will, at the very least, make you more conscious of your everyday actions and the importance of living directly in the moment, rather than stuck in the past or fretting about the future. Turning inwards and looking at yourself ultimately has a more powerful and positive effect on the world than just focusing on others.

How Not to Die by Dr Michael Greger

This is one of the easiest to read and most comprehensive books on ultimate nutrition I have come across. Foods that are good for this, foods that are good for that and ultimately foods to eat for a long and healthy life. You will learn so much about different vegetables and fruits you never knew. If you are really intent on changing your health for ever, this is a must read.

Food affects your mindset just as much as your body

If you eat processed foods every day it is likely, in fact it is certain, that it will affect your mood. Often we don't know what our optimal mood and state of being is. I'm as guilty of this as the next person. As we know, for years I ate quite badly and neglected my gut – I had no clue how much my gut dictated everything else in my body, from my mood to my attention span, my energy levels and emotions, to my metabolism.

The truth is, your brain speaks to your gut constantly. And it will sigh and roll its eyes when you eat junk food because it knows that it will not give you any kind of benefit whatsoever (OK, maybe a few minutes of enjoyment while you're eating, but then you will feel like shit afterwards). I try to remember that feeling and visualise that full, uncomfortable groggy feeling that junk food brings whenever I am tempted by it. I also visualise the feeling I get when I eat something healthy, like a massive lentil bake with sweet potato and loads of delicious flavours – my body always feels so grateful and happy, and full of energy and a positive spirit, and that feeling lasts a lot longer.

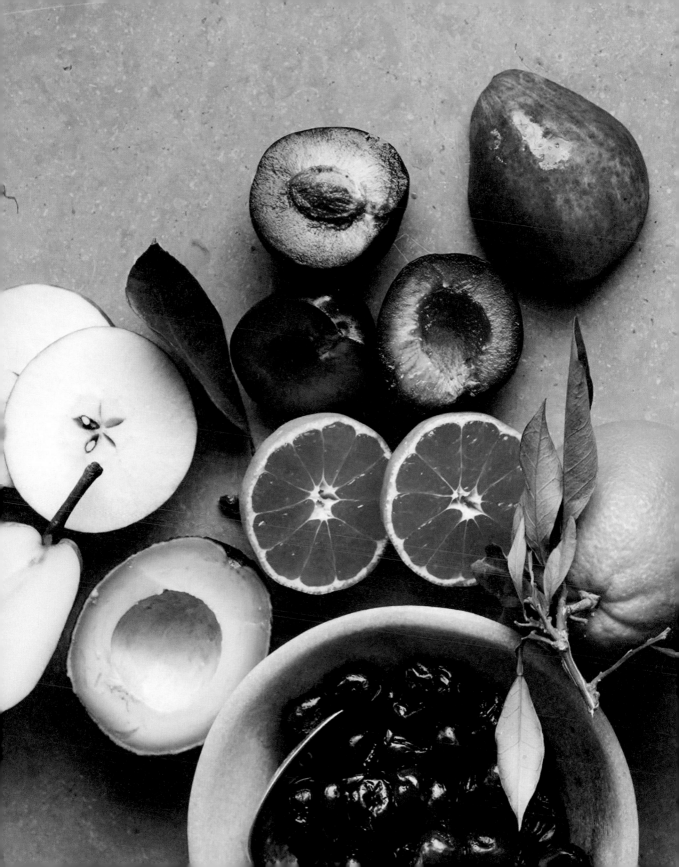

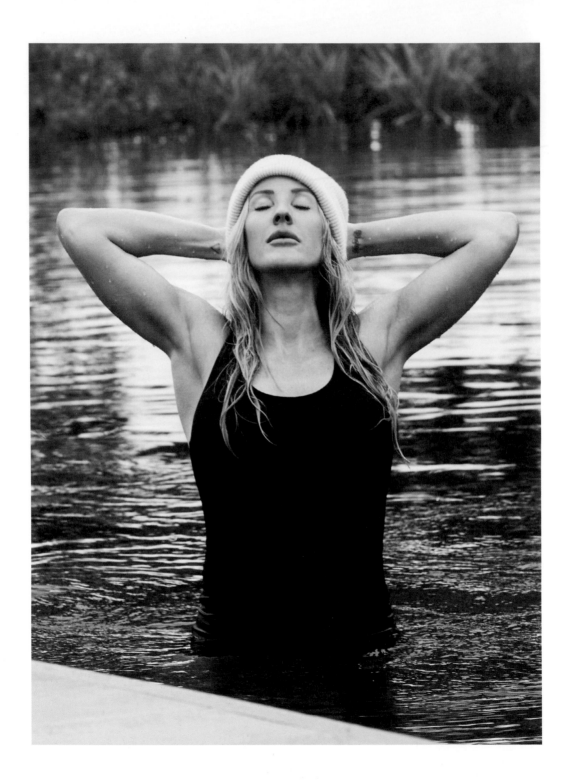

6

FIND YOUR STRENGTH

'You have to exercise, or at some point you'll just break down'

BARACK OBAMA, FORMER PRESIDENT OF THE UNITED STATES

After so many years of trial and error, of loving exercise and fitness and training, but not quite understanding how it all clicked together, now I feel I have the balance just right. I love all types of workouts and really try to mix things up, because that stops me from ever getting bored and the variation keeps me physically and mentally strong.

The beauty of boxing

One of my favourite things to do is to box, which I started doing regularly in 2015. I decided I wanted to take up boxing and was asking around for a coach when the boxing promoter Eddie Hearn told me about a former-boxer-turned-trainer called Darren Barker. Eddie suggested I go down to Darren's gym in London to meet him and from the minute we met we hit it off right away. He's been coached by some of the best coaches out there, including his dad, who was also a boxer, and he has a great way of simplifying things and making them fun. I have a lot of respect for him as a teacher and a friend.

The way I feel when I'm boxing is pretty close to how I feel when I'm on stage. No other workout comes close. I love running, doing weights, going to the gym, but boxing is, as they say, different gravy. Not only does it give all the feels, similarly to the moment I first walk out in front of that crowd, it's also given me the stamina I need to run around on that stage and perform for that crowd. It makes me feel that I can keep going for ever.

I'm going to toot my horn here – after all we've talked about that self-deprecation reflex – I am weirdly good at boxing and a bit of a natural, or so I've been told. It's my second favourite thing to do after singing and, if I wasn't a singer, as I said at the start of this book, I genuinely think I might have tried professional boxing. I go into a zone when I box: everything is up to me, and nobody can save me except myself. It requires me to be patient, unemotional, strong, quick, focused. All those things it's hard to be in real life, you have to be in boxing. On TV, especially in the later rounds, boxing looks messy and bloody. But it's a beautiful sport, full of skill and mindfulness. It's completely exhilarating and when I walk away from the boxing gym, I always feel stronger and more confident.

At one point I was training three times a week, which is pretty exhausting. You're really throwing those punches, and the next day I could hardly move. You have to use your days off to work on your posture and keeping up cardio in between sessions is absolutely key in boxing as well. At my peak I was training in the boxing gym three times a week, running three times a week and doing yoga once a week to stretch out.

It's a fantastic sport, a sport like no other, and it involves amazing skill, strength, courage and dedication. You have to be really, really good to be at the top and my boxing coach, Darren, is one of the very best.

'The way I feel when I'm boxing is pretty close to how I feel when I'm on stage'

ELLIE

Meet . . . DARREN BARKER, my boxing coach

Darren is a British former professional boxer who competed between 2004 and 2013, holding multiple titles at middleweight, including the IBF title in 2013, the Commonwealth title between 2007 and 2009 and the British title in 2009. As an amateur, Darren represented England at the 2002 Commonwealth Games and won a gold medal in the light-welterweight division.

Ellie: How did you first get into boxing?

Darren: 'I can't remember a life without boxing. Growing up in Barnet, North London, my dad, Terry, was a top amateur boxer, winning the ABA title in 1980, which is the best thing you can win as an amateur in this country. But there was no money in amateur boxing back in the 1970s and 80s, so he earned his living as a hod carrier, lugging bricks around a building site.

'As a kid, I remember my mum would put all his trophies out on display, but my dad is the most modest man you'll ever meet and he didn't like any fuss being made over his achievements. Growing up, we watched boxing together all the time and we were always messing about and sparring in the kitchen. However, my dad never pushed me into boxing and would have been happy with whatever path I took. But when I was eleven, I took myself down to Finchley Boxing Club, which was a 10-minute bus ride away from our house, and that's where I learned the basics of boxing. The rest is history.'

Ellie: So you've been boxing ever since you were a kid?

Darren: 'Yes! After a few years at the Finchley Boxing Club, I left to join Repton Boxing Club in Bethnal Green. Without being disrespectful to Finchley, it was like leaving a small primary school and going straight to a top university. I was so star-struck by the fighters down there, some of whom went on to be Olympic gold medallists. The club had something about it. It lit a fire in me. All I remember thinking was that I didn't want to be the worst one down there. So I trained really hard. I loved it.'

Ellie: Boxing is one of my favourite ways to train. Can you tell me more about why it is so good for you?

Darren: 'As a cardio sport, nothing really beats boxing because it uses practically every single muscle in your body: your core, your shoulders, right the way down to your feet. You're on your toes and on the go the whole time. It's fun and it's tough, but best of all it's also a mental sport. It releases feel-good endorphins and it's a brilliant stress release. You can take out a bad day on a punchbag.'

Ellie: It is often seen as quite a male sport, but boxing is good for everybody, right?

Darren: 'Yes. You're a brilliant boxer! You can punch hard and you've got this fiery passion for boxing, which is great to see. Put it this way, I wouldn't want to fight you!

'I also think boxing is a good sport for children and teenagers, both boys and girls. Boxing teaches you about discipline and respect. It teaches you how to control your aggression and how to work as part of a team. When I was growing up, I had such a sense of pride belonging to my club and representing it with my fellow boxers and teammates. There was a sense of camaraderie among us. I had a brilliant family and home life, but not all kids have that at home and boxing clubs can offer those youngsters a sense of belonging.'

Ellie: Why did you decide to take up coaching?

> *Darren:* 'I've been coached by some of the best coaches out there, including my dad, and they've always had a great way of simplifying instructions and not over-complicating things. I tried to transfer that into my coaching.'

Ellie: You've always told me that boxing is as much of a mental sport as a physical one. Could you tell me a bit more about that?

> *Darren:* 'As well as keeping you fit, boxing keeps you on your toes mentally because you have to constantly be alert. If you lose focus or your mind wanders, even for a few seconds, then bam, it's game over in the blink of an eye. When you're boxing your mind is on boxing, nothing else; not your inbox or your to-do list. It's only when you come away from a boxing session that you realise how focused you've been and how good that is for your mind.
>
> 'It also drives you to train hard. When I was boxing professionally, I used to always imagine my opponent was training harder than me, which made me want to work twice as hard.'

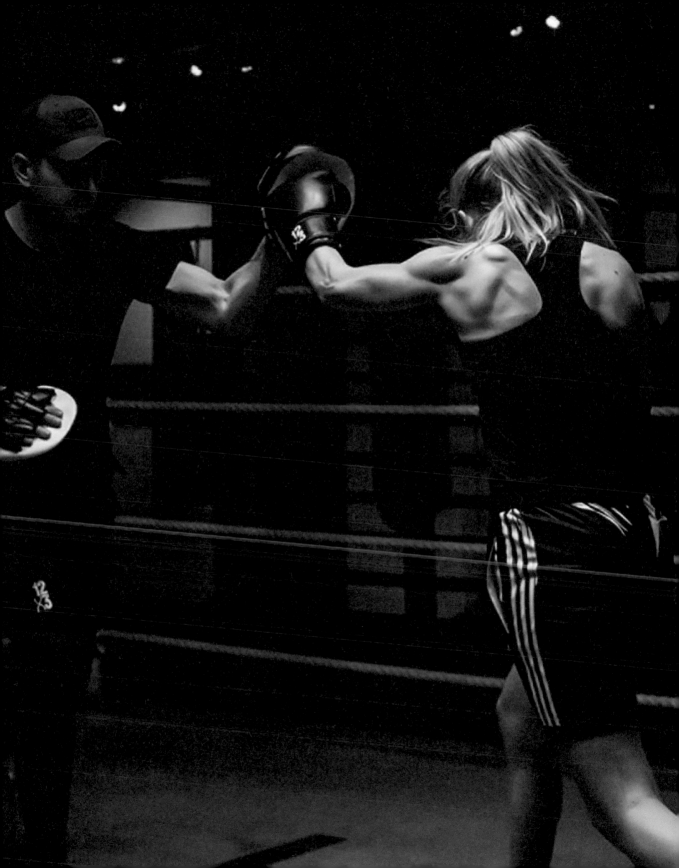

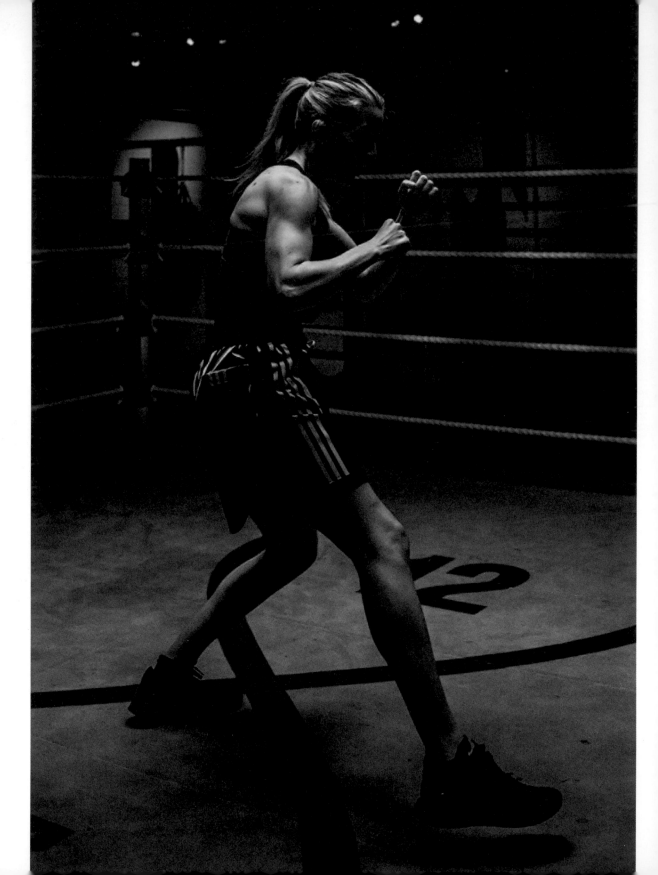

What is your core and why is boxing so good for it?

BY DARREN BARKER

'Your core is a complex set of muscles that are located deep within your trunk. It is made up of several muscles and extends far beyond just your six-pack – and we shouldn't just rely on sit-ups to work it.

'Having a strong and healthy core is more than just having a flat stomach. A strong core gives you better balance and posture and helps reduce back pain. If you work on your core you're also less likely to get injured from a workout, and even the bends and lifts of daily life. It's the centre of all movement.

'Boxing engages all of your core muscles, including your rectus abdominis (basically your "abs"), the internal and external obliques (the muscle on either side of your abdomen), erector spinae (a set of muscles in your lower back) and your transverse abdominis (the deep, internal core muscles that wrap around your sides and spine).

'All the twists, jabs and bends of boxing keep your core engaged, fired up and strong. As you throw a shot towards a punchbag, or your partner's boxing pads, you have to engage your core muscles. So alongside sparring, I do a lot of core work with my clients, including the ones I've shared with you later in this book.

'However, I still think the very best core exercise around is the good old-fashioned plank. I used to try and outdo my boxing teammates all the time by holding the longest plank. My record is about 8 minutes.'

HOW TO DO THE PERFECT PLANK

'First get into a forearm plank position, with your elbows and forearms on the ground underneath your shoulders. Your elbows should be under your shoulders and your feet should be hip-width apart.

'Now push up and hold yourself up by your toes and forearms. Ensure your body is in a straight line, with your back straight and your head and neck in a neutral position. Don't look down or lower your head, because it will be extra weight.

'Keep your core engaged, imagining yourself pulling in your belly button. Don't hold your breath. Keep breathing; inhale through your nose and exhale through your mouth. You shouldn't feel pain in your lower back – this move works your core, not your back. If you feel it in your lower back, it means your core isn't properly engaged, so reset and rethink your form before trying again.

'If you're new to fitness, aim to hold this position for 30 seconds at a time, building up gradually to 1 minute each time.'

HOW NOT TO WEAR YOUR BODY OUT WITH BOXING

'I'm a great example of how boxing can add a lot of wear and tear to your body. I've had to have two hip operations, which my doctor said was either due to a birth defect or wear and tear from sport. I'm guessing it's the latter.

'The old tried and tested method of staying fit for boxing was to pound the roads and just do miles and miles of running. That's what my dad's generation did, and the one before them, but because of my hip operation I couldn't do that level of running. But I still needed to keep my base level of fitness and stamina to be able to box, so I had to find substitutes. First, I started swimming, which I found just as hard work as running but much gentler on my joints. Then I began to incorporate some extra training into it, with underwater punching for resistance. I would do straight punching in the water for 3 minutes.

'Then, for my last five contests, I did yoga alongside boxing, which I think helped me win the world title. My first attempt to win the title ended in defeat, and then I took up yoga and won. Yoga increased my speed and agility. It's really good for joints and flexibility, but it definitely made me stronger as well. The old-school mentality with boxing is to run and run until you're knackered, but the newer coaches coming through are reading up on the sports science that shows strength and conditioning from things like swimming, stretching, yoga and walking really help, too. I often do a little yoga routine in the morning, to keep me fit, but also to help my mindset and stress levels.

'So if you do take up boxing – either with a coach, or a group boxing class at your local gym – make sure to mix it up with some other, gentler workouts. They'll help you prevent injury, as well as making you a better boxer. In fact, this is true of any exercise. By mixing up your workouts, you give overused muscles and joints some time to rest and recover before putting them to work again.'

Why every woman should give boxing a try

BY KATIE TAYLOR

Katie Taylor is a professional boxer, two-weight world champion and the current undisputed lightweight champion. She was born in Ireland and has been credited with raising the profile of women's boxing around the world. She was also the flag bearer for Ireland at the 2012 London Olympics opening ceremony, the games where she went on to win an Olympic gold medal in the lightweight division.

'My dad was a boxer and some of my earliest memories are of him shadow-boxing or skipping in our tiny kitchen, or hitting the punchbag in the makeshift gym he built in our back garden. My mum was also a boxing judge (the first female to judge in our national stadium in fact). So I guess it was never a foreign or male sport to me. I was exposed to it from the very beginning.

'I was very athletic as a young girl and I loved all kinds of sports, from football and running to basketball, karate and even table tennis. It was karate that was mainly responsible for me taking up boxing competitively. From the age of about nine, I was getting serious about karate and started attending competitions, but apparently non-contact combat sports didn't suit me; I was disqualified from the girls' competition for being a bit too enthusiastic with my punches!

'This led to me being entered me into the boys' competition, but then I was disqualified again for the same thing. So my dad took me to our local boxing club with him and that solved that problem; and it has been my life's passion ever since.

'I just love everything about boxing. I love the honesty of standing in front of your opponent and looking them right in the eye. I love the respect between the two fighters who have shared a ring together; it is a fellowship of blood, sweat and tears. I love the feeling of a boxing gym; the smell and the atmosphere is a heady mix of hardships and heartaches and dreams and aspirations. It feels like an escape, an oasis from all the complications of the outside world.

'I love the qualities that boxing rewards: hard work, dedication, courage, strength, technical skill, respect, ambition. I love the questions boxing asks of your character. It demands an answer to the question "Do you have what it takes?" And what it takes is found in the depths of your soul.

'From a fitness point of view, there's no better motivator to move than to stop getting punched in the face! The ring is a punishing place for those who take shortcuts in the gym. But even for those who will never step into a ring for a competitive fight, boxing is one of best ways to get in shape. Every time you throw a punch, you are demanding something from every muscle in your body, from your toes through to your hips and torso, right up through your shoulders and arms.

'Punching with the correct technique is very tiring; it requires an explosive contraction of hundreds of muscles. It's also a very complete fitness regime since it places a huge demand on your cardio, strength, strength endurance, speed and agility. Anybody who has punched a bag full throttle for one minute will know what I'm talking about.

'And then, of course, there are the mental-health benefits. Exercise of any type is known to be very good for mental health and reducing stress. It is hard to pinpoint exactly why boxing seems to be a particularly good stress reducer. I think one reason is because punching a bag can release tension that is building from frustration over a situation. I couldn't imagine cycling or jogging could have the same impact as boxing when it comes to getting that frustration out.

'The other theory I have is that there is a kind of rhythm to boxing that is therapeutic. You hear it when someone is hitting a bag or hitting pads; there's a musicality to the "thwack" sound, the combinations and flurries of punches. I find that very soothing.

'The other thing about mental health is that we need both a strong connection to ourselves and to others to have healthy minds. Team sports are a great way to build connections with others. But boxing is an individual sport and I have always found it a great place to let my thoughts and emotions breathe. Punching my bag in my basement on a Sunday evening with my favourite music playing in the background can sometimes be a spiritual moment.

'Boxing also teaches you respect for yourself and for others. You often hear boxers "trash talk" each other before fights and you might think they have no respect for each other. This is usually a gimmick to promote the fight. Almost always, when the final bell rings, the real heartfelt respect and honour is evident between them. But boxing is also a great tool for developing self-respect and self-confidence. Walking into a boxing gym is an intimidating prospect for most, so even taking that step takes enough courage to warrant holding your head up high. Even more so for anyone who dares to step between the ropes.

'Anyone who has done so will tell you that it takes guts, real guts. And as you stick it out, your progress will be tangible and you will grow in self-confidence, which has a way of spilling out into other areas of your life.

'Why should women try boxing? Because they have two hands, just like men! Boxing is not about being aggressive. It is about self-control, self-belief, poise, strength, courage, technique, resilience, focus and ambition. Many of the women I know have these qualities in spades.

'When it comes to getting started with boxing, as with anything, the first step forwards is the hardest. In this case, the first step is getting yourself down to your local boxing gym. The local gym is the heartbeat of the sport. It is a daunting prospect to step through those doors for the first time and I think it takes even more courage if you are female since boxing gyms are so heavily male-dominated.

'But taking that step is the hardest. Once you're in, you will fall in love with the sounds and the vibrancy of the room. You will find something noble in the middle of all the madness that makes you want to come back. And there starts a lifelong passion for the beautiful science.'

Three things I always tell myself when I am struggling to find the motivation to exercise

1. Physical exercise brings mental and physical benefits. Exercise doesn't just affect your body, it also impacts the way you think, the decisions you make and the way you respond to situations.

2. You are supposed to be fit and healthy and function well. But you have to give your body and mind what it needs to reach your fullest potential, both emotionally and physically.

3. Being uncomfortable makes you stronger. Maybe try a slightly longer run or a different workout. Or perhaps try having a cold shower to raise your tolerance to cold water.

'Exercise is a celebration of what your body can do. Not a punishment for what you ate.'

KEVIN NG, YOGA AND MINDFULNESS COACH

The joys of wild exercise

I recently did an eight-mile hike uphill in the Lake District. The sideways rain blew in all directions, soaking us through, but all around were other people doing the very same thing, unbothered. I saw people in their seventies right down to little kids, wrapped up in raincoats and walking boots, who were clearly more used to the hills than I was.

I was completely out of breath and looking like a drowned rat, but the combination of sweaty, heart-pumping exercise and being outside in nature, with the uneven ground beneath my feet keeping my core engaged, and the patchwork of greens and browns never-ending, was an absolute tonic.

I got such a thrill from the hike, I decided to do a fell run, which is sometimes known as hill running and involves running off-road in the countryside, often uphill. The name comes from the fells (mountain ranges) of northern Britain, especially those in the Lake District. It makes a thrilling change from running on the treadmill because you get different scenery every few minutes, you can go at your own pace on the different inclines, and the different surfaces force your body to work harder to keep you upright, which fires up all your muscles.

When you're fell running you have to use your whole body, especially your mind, which has to focus on the ever-changing terrain. Sometimes you go slow, on the inclines or over the rocky patches, and other times you add in some sprints on the flat surfaces or when you go downhill, making it a great HIIT workout, too.

You don't have to run if you don't want to. You could try walking in an area with some steep hills, walking to the top of a tall hill and down again, taking in the views. It's so immensely good for you, and if you go alone you can listen to a good podcast while you're at it.

Taking the plunge: why I'm a cold-water swimming convert

A couple of years ago I was reluctantly at a house party in Scotland with my husband and some of his friends (it was a particularly socially anxious time for me). Next to the house was a loch, the kind that you can just tell from the rich, dark green of the water is bloody cold; warm water doesn't look like that. It was both monstrous and majestic. I was so intrigued. I was always scared of jumping into water when I was a kid. It didn't seem remotely natural to do so. I'm also always the person wearing three or four layers on a cold day, standing there with the hairdryer on, trying to warm up. Even now I'm always cold after coming home from a run. (I have Raynaud's disease too, which affects the circulation of blood to your hands and feet and means they can quickly become incredibly cold and blue or white.) But as I've got older, I've realised the fear of doing something is often far worse than the reality of it.

So, back to the house party. There I was, when some of Caspar's beautiful, fit and tanned friends suggested jumping into the icy lake next to the house. I really didn't want to do it but there was a bit of light-hearted peer pressure going on and, not wanting to look like a loser, I took the leap. It was as cold as it looked – painfully so – and I hated every one of them for making me do it. It was only afterwards that I admitted to myself how good and invincible it made me feel, and within days my anxiety cleared up as well.

After that, I couldn't help researching the benefits of cold-water immersion and I've slowly got myself used to cold-water swimming. Studies have found it's really good for the immune system. It's proven to help you sleep better and can help lift depressive symptoms. Research that came out in 2020 also showed regular cold-water swimmers are less likely to suffer from dementia. And scientists at Cambridge University found a 'cold shock' protein can help slow down degenerative diseases like Alzheimer's.

I'm not surprised wild swimming has so many positive effects on the brain because even a 10-minute swim leaves you feeling euphoric. It's been steadily getting more popular in the last few years, with millions of us in the UK heading for lakes or outdoor pools every year. At the time of writing this, my friend Fearne Cotton has been posting about the 'pure exhilaration' she feels swimming in the sea in autumn and the benefits of cold-water therapy in general. When lockdown happened and gyms were closed, even more people swam outside, and Instagram is full of increasing numbers of us swimming in misty lakes and icy lidos.

Jumping in – as I did at the Scottish house party – is definitely not advised, however. *Face palm*. Instead, you should walk in slowly, submerging your skin bit by bit (especially in the winter months) so you don't get that cold-water shock where your skin feels like it's on fire and your heart rate goes through the roof. Go in nice and steady and fight the urge to head straight back to shore – or the side of the pool if you're at an open-air lido – because that initial feeling of cold and 'Why on earth am I doing this?' will pass, I promise. Soon your body will adjust, and you'll start to feel refreshed and energised. I'm now a complete convert. There is nothing as special as swimming in the sea, or in a cold, clear, deep lake, surrounded by trees, and watching birds land on the water a few feet away from where you're swimming. I talked earlier about the healing power of nature – and the fact that spending time in forests and green space has been shown to lift our mood and strengthen our immune system – and escaping into cold water is another, brilliant, invigorating version of this.

And it's also great for our mental health. As you enter the water and spend the first minute or so trying to catch your breath and regulating your breathing, the shock of the cold water sweeping across your body clears your mind of anything that's troubling it. Endorphins are pumped out and you will feel calm, capable and happy. And I promise you, by the time you get back to shore, you'll be feeling pretty epic and wondering when you can go again.

'If you move your body every single day to help you do something you love, like dancing or hiking, or wild swimming, you will love your body for what it allows you to do, not for what it looks like. And because you need your body's help to do those things, you'll treat it well and appreciate it for the strong and beautiful thing it is.'

ELLIE

HOW TO STAY SAFE WHILE WILD SWIMMING

If you're in the UK, look at the RNLI's safety advice around rip currents and details of low and high tides. Swim at either a lido, an open-water facility that's staffed, or go with a friend. Never go wild swimming alone, unless you're very experienced and people know where you are.

- No matter what time of year you're swimming, and especially between September and March, never underestimate the temperature of the water. Even when it's sunny outside, always walk into the water slowly, going under the water bit by bit, to give your body a chance to acclimatise. If you jump in too quickly, the 'cold-shock response' can cause you to gasp, which not only affects your breath control (vital for swimming, and especially wild swimming) but could also cause you to take a gulp of water, which could be dangerous if the water isn't clean enough to drink.

- Plan for when you get out, which is when you'll be at your coldest. Take a large towel to dry off, take off your wetsuit or swimming costume immediately, and change into warm, dry layers. Dryrobes, which are changing robes, are particularly good for helping you keep warm and covered up while you're getting changed. Whether you're swimming in autumn or winter, take gloves and a woolly hat, and a flask of hot water or tea.

- Don't spend too long in the water if you're new to it. Build up your tolerance by adding a blast of cold water to your daily showers. Start with 30–60 seconds, before slowly building to a few minutes. As muscles get cold in the water, they can become stiff, tired and clumsy. Keep your routes short at first and stay close to the shore – you can always repeat a loop. Having said that, keep at it. The more you do it, the easier

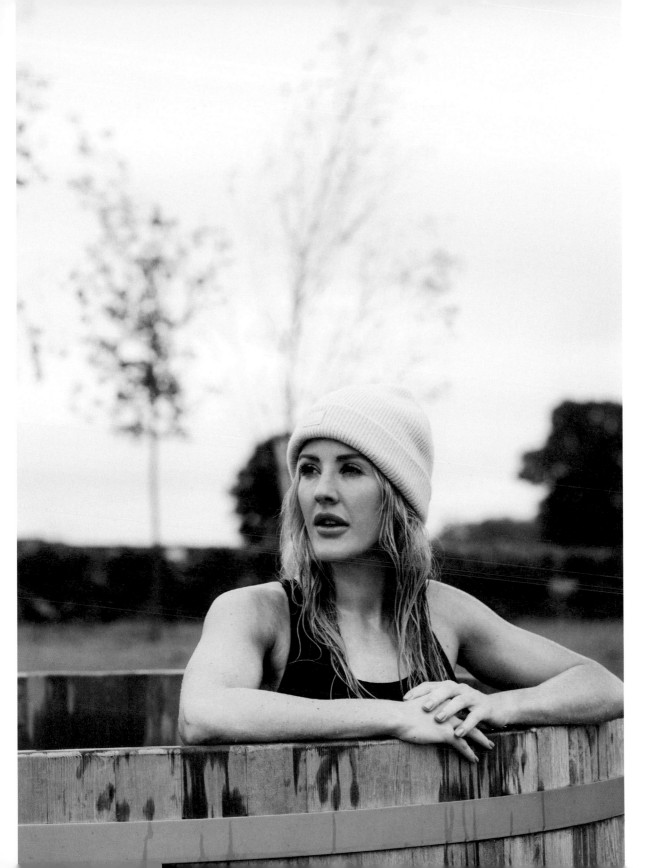

it will become. If you're pregnant, speak to your GP before swimming in cold water.

- Finally, check out www.wildswim.com, a worldwide free swim map, or follow @theoutdoorswimmingsociety on Instagram, a worldwide community of outdoor swimmers.

ESSENTIAL KIT FOR WILD SWIMMING

Wetsuit: Some wild swimmers like going in the water in their swimming costumes or trunks, but I'd suggest you use a wetsuit in the colder months. Some triathlon swimmers swear by them for helping them to glide through the water and shave time off their swim.

Surf suit: These are like high-necked, long-sleeved swimming costumes. They're great for spring or autumn swims because, while not keeping you as warm as a wetsuit, they'll keep your chest and arms warm.

Swim socks: These are advisable in very cold water and also to protect your feet if you're swimming in lakes with pebbly or rocky beds.

Swim gloves: These are good to keep your hands (which are an extremity and get colder quicker) warm in very cold temperatures.

A woolly hat: If you swim between October and March, you may want to wear a woolly bobble hat to keep your head warm. This only works if you keep your head above water and do breaststroke. Otherwise, a woolly hat is a must for when you get out because that's when you'll lose a lot of heat from your head.

Meet . . . CATIE MILLER, my barre teacher

Catie Miller is my barre teacher and founder of OONA Series (www.oonaseries.com, @oonaseries). Barre is a combination of ballet and Pilates. I was introduced to it by the designer Alice Temperley, who is also a client of Catie's.

Ellie: Can you tell everybody a little bit about barre? What is it?

Catie: 'Barre is a workout technique that's a fusion of ballet and Pilates, with cardio thrown in as well. It's focused on low-weight but high-intensity and high-frequency movements.'

Ellie: How did you get into it?

Catie: 'I'm originally from Albuquerque, New Mexico, in the USA, and I grew up dancing. I come from a dance family, and as a child I did everything from ballet to jazz and modern dance. I travelled all over the USA competing and even got to work with Mia Michaels, who is a legend in the dance world. She's worked with Madonna, Prince and Gloria Estefan.

'I loved the discipline that dance instilled in me. I had to show up to dance class on time, no holes in my tights my hair sprayed just so. When I walked into that room, I had to be fully present. Dancing has instilled so many life skills within me that I have weaved into many aspects of my life, from motherhood to business and beyond.'

Ellie: What brought you to London?

Catie: 'I met my husband in 2009 and moved across the pond to join him. Once in London, everything was so new and exciting but there was a sense of connection that I felt was missing. As soon as I stepped into a few dance classes at London's Pineapple Dance Studio it fuelled my soul like crazy!

'I became pregnant with my first son and one day wandered into a local barre class. I looked around the room and there was an incredibly strong woman in one corner flowing through the workout, a man in another corner and also a pregnant woman just like me. The diversity in this space is incredible, I thought. I remember walking home after the class and saying to my husband, "This is what I'm going to do. I'm going to open a studio." I wanted to pair my love of movement with my love of community.'

Ellie: What then?

Catie: 'I dug into my dancing roots, went on lots of courses and opened up a pop-up studio in Mayfair, London. The plan was to run it for three months, but it ended up staying open for two years.

Then we opened a studio in the heart of Marylebone on the High Street which created incredible demand and exposure. Then in 2020 we launched a virtual well-being space called Oona Series where we not only teach virtual workout classes but offer on demand sessions as well as holistic conversations and workshops around the topics of physical, mental and social well-being. It has truly been a humbling experience knowing that no matter where we are in the world we can move, find connection and seek tools to help us live a more joyful and fulfilling life.'

Ellie: In our sessions you talk to me a lot about the importance of breathwork. Can you tell me more about that?

Catie: 'It's important to be aware of when to inhale and exhale with barre – and with all exercise really. When we inhale, our body relaxes, and our heart rate lowers. So you should exhale on the effort, as you engage your abdomen to protect and support your spine. Proper breathwork pairs mind and body to movement, and when you learn to breathe properly you engage all your muscles. Barre classes teach you how to control this.

Ellie: What are the other benefits of barre?

Catie: 'Barre is a great de-stressor. I have a lot of clients who are parents, or working in law or finance, and they walk into my class and I can see they're already thinking about something else.

'Their mind is racing through their to-do list and I can spot it a mile off. My challenge is to get them to be fully present in the room, so I tell them to shake off their stress, leave everything at the door, and focus on themselves for 45 minutes. Because they're having to follow all my instructions – "do a plié (a word most of us haven't heard since we were four), inhale, exhale, lift" – they don't have time to let their minds wander.'

Ellie: It's a tough workout though, right?

Catie: 'Absolutely! During our first session I remember you setting your fitness tracker to yoga mode and I said, no, set it to the HIIT function. Despite ballet's gentle reputation, a performance is very similar to a HIIT class. Ballerinas build their endurance on stage, they have moments of peaking heart rate as they push through their performance, and then they stop and let their heart rate come down. Ballerinas are some of the fittest athletes around and they need serious stamina to perform. My workouts last for 45 minutes and they're full on.

'When we first started working together, I think the biggest surprise for you was how much it got your heart rate up. After the warm-up, I remember we started what I call the deep sculpt, and you picked up these tiny hand weights and were like, "Really?" You were used to lifting really heavy weights. And I said, "Trust me, after 2 minutes your arms are going to be burning and screaming." Ten minutes of not dropping your arm later and you realised what I meant! Barre works those tiny little muscles that haven't been used for a long time. That's when the sculpting and lengthening happens.'

Ellie: Caspar has done one of your classes, too!

Catie: 'Yes, I remember we were doing an early morning class one day and he asked if he could join in. He said, "So this is going to be a nice gentle stretch, right?" I said, "Not really, but give it a go."

'I think he was planning on doing another bootcamp class later that day. But when we finished the class, all dripping in sweat, he said, "OK, I'm not going to the other class now." I think it blew his mind!'

The power of breath

BY CATIE MILLER

'Happiness is moving, getting ready for change and loving it'
BONIFACE VERNEY-CARRON, OSTEOPATH AND CO-FOUNDER OONA SERIES

'Never underestimate the power of your breath. Focused breathwork has not only connected me deeper to my workouts and provided greater physical results, it has also carried me through life.'

'The quote above from Boniface, one of my mentors, made me reflect on the importance of a positive mindset. I talk to my clients a lot about setting these intentions at the beginning of each workout because it is in these moments that we need to dig deep, calm our mind and focus on our breath.

'Here are five simple breathing exercises you can do at home every day. Grab a mat, put on your favourite playlist and your cosy socks, and settle into the rhythm of your breath.'

BREATH MOVE 1

'Lying on your back, let the legs relax into whatever position they wish. You can lie straight-legged, knees bent or soles of the feet together.

'Closing your eyes, place your hands on your rib cage and start breathing in through the nose and out of the mouth. Think about taking long deep inhalations to fill the lungs and let your ribcage open up and out into your hands. I like to imagine the rhythm of waves, matching my breath to the tide.

'The longer you can draw the breathwork in and out, the deeper sense of "reset" you achieve.

'Start to scan your body from the crown of your head all the way down to your toes – think about softening your eyes, jaw, chest, belly, hips, glutes and feet. As soon as your mind starts to wander (which is normal), bring it back to the rhythm of the waves. This is a practice and something we need to do daily to train the mind and body towards discipline.

'**Tip:** Try this technique throughout your day during any moments where you feel your mind wandering, stressed or heavy within your thoughts. Intentional breathing helps to shift and align our senses, leading to a feeling of self-support and calmness.'

BREATH MOVE 2

'Staying on your back, hug your knees into your chest and lower them with control to one side. Keeping your knees together, reach your arms out from your shoulders into a "T" position and gaze over the opposite shoulder to the direction your knees are now in.

'Taking your focus back to your intentional breathing, think about relaxing your shoulder blades onto the mat, deepening the mid-spine twist with each exhale. Close your eyes and continue breathing for 5–10 long, connected inhales and exhalations.

'Slowly bring your legs through to the centre using your core and then gently lower them to the opposite side and repeat.

'**Tip:** Gently press one hand down into the top knee to deepen the stretch.'

BREATH MOVE 3

'Lying on your back with your legs extended along the mat, draw one knee into your chest and gently move your hip around the socket, creating four to eight big circles in each direction.

'Once finished, unfold your leg up to the ceiling while holding behind your calf or hamstring (avoid holding behind the knee). Focus on lengthening through the back of your leg while pointing and flexing your foot to create a deeper stretch through your hamstrings and calf muscles.

'Gently bend your knee, place your foot back on the mat, and repeat on the other side.

'**Tip:** Remember to focus on the rhythm of your breath when circling your knee and hip in its socket. Think long, even breaths while ensuring both hips stay in line and your pelvis stays in neutral.'

BREATH MOVE 4

'Starting in a cross-legged seated position, bend one leg and extend the other leg to the side with your knee pointing upwards. Reaching your opposite arm up and over your head towards the leg that is extended, focus on breathing into the side of your ribcage while feeling the gentle stretch through the side of your body. You can rest the other arm behind the extended leg with your elbow gently pressing into the floor. Hold the stretch for five to ten long, even breaths.

'Sit up straight, restack your spine and then repeat on the other side.

'**Tip:** Flip your palm upwards for the final few breaths to deepen the stretch and add a gentle spine rotation. Continue the breath pattern of breathing in through the nose and out of the mouth while ensuring both sitting bones stay down on the mat.'

BREATH MOVE 5

'Starting on all fours, with a neutral neck, spine and pelvis, press your palms into the mat, gently moving from a cat to cow position*, focusing all the time on moving with your breath.

'Enjoy the stretch across your upper back as well as feeling the length through your abdominals. Work on articulating through each vertebra, creating space and length through your spine.

'Repeat this movement four to eight times, before returning to a neutral spine. Once complete, press your bottom back to your heels and relax into a child's pose position. Finish the way you started by gently closing your eyes and breathing long, even breaths in through your nose and out of your mouth. Scan your body, melting your forehead into the mat, whilst gently rocking the hips from side to side.

'**Tip:** Think about your mid-spine lifting up as you press through the palms during your cat position. Initiate the roll from your tailbone as you gently move into the cow stretch and soften the elbows as you do.'

*HOW TO DO THE CAT–COW MOVE

'Get on all fours with your hands beneath your shoulders and your knees beneath your hips. Keep your back in a neutral position. Inhale for the "cow" position – tilt your pelvis back so your tailbone sticks up, let your belly drop down, relax and gaze up towards the ceiling.

'Next, exhale and come into the "cat" position. Arch your back slightly, allowing your head to drop and your bottom to stick up and out. Pull your belly button into your spine and keep your abs engaged. Allow your head to drop down, so your back is making a "C" shape. Keep your arms pushed into the mat, and your belly button pulled in. This is the cat position.'

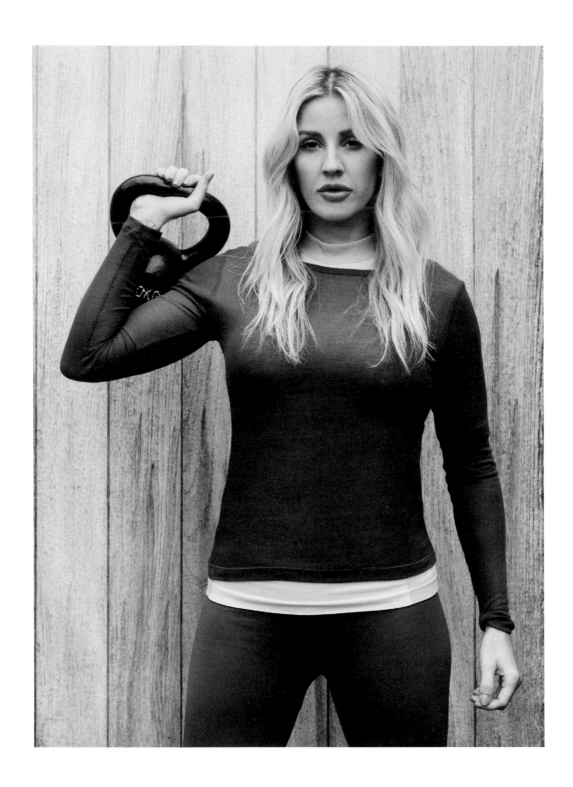

7

HOW I MOVE: The Workouts

Your body is designed to run, swim, move, stretch and exercise. It's not supposed to sit still for long periods, behind a laptop or on a sofa binge-watching Netflix, or hunched over a phone. Those things are fine in small doses, but we need to move.

In the previous chapters I talked about the importance of movement and the types of exercises I've tried over the years. In this chapter, three of my favourite trainers are going to give you a workout to try.

They're all from different walks of fitness life. Matt Roberts is my personal trainer, and he's going to talk you through five home-based workouts he's designed, each tailored to a different time of day or energy level. Darren Barker is my boxing coach, and his box-fit workout is the same one his dad did to get fit before boxing matches in the 1970s. And finally, Catie Miller, my brilliant barre teacher, is going to talk you through a full-body barre warm-up and sculpt class (a workout inspired by ballet, yoga and Pilates).

They're all very different types of movement and, as I said in chapter one, this book isn't prescriptive, so pick and choose which ones you want to do and when. They are all brilliant workouts that will keep you fit, healthy, sculpted, lean and energised. Enjoy them . . . (I always do!)

Meet . . . MATT ROBERTS, my personal trainer

Matt is my personal trainer, who I see around three times a week when I'm in London.

Ellie: Can you tell me a bit about how you approach training plans for your clients? What would a perfect week of training look like?

Matt: 'No exercise week can ever be fully expected to deliver on perfection. It can aim to do so, and it can occasionally happen or come close, but the reality is that we are all different and we all have to cope with whatever life, our body, our mind and the world throws at us on an hour-by-hour and day-by-day basis.

'It's a given that we are going to aim for perfection of a sort. Naturally. However, what that perfection looks like varies from person to person enormously. For some, the goal is to be super-lean, for some to be stronger and for some to remain the same. There are sporting goals, achievement-based objectives (climb that mountain, swim that sea, do that 10k), and then there are objectives that are emotional and also hugely important ("I want to feel more positive and energised" or "I sleep and perform better when I've been exercising consistently"). Exercise and wellbeing has never been a one size fits all, never will be, and the more we learn about science and ourselves, the more that is being proven on an amazing scale.

Ellie: That makes sense. Is there anything else that impacts the way you plan programmes for your clients? For example, does my career effect the workouts you plan for me?

Matt: 'Absolutely. You're a performer; an artist and a public figure in a world that demands more and scrutinises on a micro level more intensely than ever. With the time, energy

169

and public perception demands come the expected days of high and low energy, as a result. By the way, this is anything but unusual, we all get this, it's just magnified when the public eye is there to remind you. It takes great focus to stay, well, focused! Footballers have problems with days when they don't train or play matches, as the highs are so high that the energy down is invariably low. As an artist you get this, too, the main difference being that you don't tend to perform twice per week or train in your art form every day, as footballers and other sportspeople do, to scratch the itch.

'Therefore the programme that I work on with you is very much a perfection-based plan (because that's just how we roll!), but one that is collaboratively constructed, based on how each day and each week shapes up and impacts on your sleep, energy or focus. And it's my job to make sure you're physically 100 per cent of what your body needs at that point in time and in the context of the overall programme goal.'

Ellie: That sounds complicated!

Matt: 'It is and it isn't. The key is to have one main programme with its constituent parts that need to be achieved (varied cardio goals, shape and strength goals and a balanced, mobile body structure) and to adapt the elements that could potentially slow down our progress by over-exhausting the system at the wrong times. It's these sessions that require the greatest care and diligence to implement at the right time and ensure we don't just go hell for leather because someone feels like letting rip!'

The elements

BY MATT ROBERTS

CARDIOVASCULAR TRAINING

'I don't think that many people have an exercise objective to just be really, really good at a Versa Climber in the gym (and if you do, you really need to take a long hard look at your personal goals). Cardio training in a gym or circuit-training environment is a means to an end. It's a brilliant one, but that's what it is.

'Ellie actually likes to amp it up on the cardio machines to test and push herself when we train, but our objective is to create a body that is able to be put to great use elsewhere. Ellie really likes to have an ambitious objective: running up a mountain, boxing in a ring (not the "boxercise" you might be thinking, I mean REAL boxing), jumping on a bike and completing a massive route. It is these types of things that should be your cardiovascular objectives. Your gym work is the tool rather than the prize.

'We are outdoor animals and we are competitive, so let's not just sit on a stationary bike going nowhere and watch TV. That is not Ellie's style and it shouldn't be yours either.

'The tools, however, do include using treadmills, ski-ergo, rowing machines, sled pushing, skipping and a whole load of other methods. Ellie uses these predominantly for High Intensity Interval Training, sessions that lasts for bursts of 20–60 seconds maximum, with rest periods that are dictated by her recovery rate.

'In intensity terms, Ellie is reaching 90–95 per cent of her maximum heart rate with her cardio training, which means hitting levels up in the 180s and 190s at times. Because Ellie and I are data nerds, we also know her HRV (Heart Rate Variability is the varied gaps between beats of the heart; the greater the variance, the higher the parasympathetic nervous system can cope, i.e. you are rested and ready to rock!), which gives a good indication of her readiness for this level of intensity on any given day.

'To see real improvement, the cardio system needs to be beaten up a little bit every other day, to a pretty vigorous degree. For Ellie, this typically happens on the days in the gym and when she goes to a circuit-training class. On another one or two days a week Ellie will build in some time for running; these are our "steady days". Now, given free reign and a goal to shoot for, Ellie would run a half-marathon just for the hell of it. This is great, but my job is to make sure we also focus on achieving our objectives, which generally means not allowing too high a frequency of long-duration cardio (more than an hour) unless there is a specific goal related to it. Ellie will usually do 5–10km runs on the "steady days", with her pace varied to reflect our bigger objective.'

STRENGTH TRAINING

'Ellie's goal with strength is to build muscle mass and high definition without the size. The truth is that it is very, very hard for women to actually build muscle mass. However, that doesn't mean that it can't or doesn't happen. Our strength programme is geared around maxing out on strength, creating muscular endurance and making sure that the whole body is in balance aesthetically and structurally.

'Any sport that we play produces subtle differences in our body posture and shape if practised enough. Think of tennis players with a much bigger forearm side than their backhand side. With Ellie, it's boxing. Boxing stance is forward and rounded (like an office worker, just with more peril!), so with our training we need to work on keeping the stance neutral and upright, and strengthening the areas of the middle back and shoulders that are dragged forwards with her boxing.

'This routine is a mixture of heavy lifting using low reps (four to six per exercise), medium resistance using systems such as supersetting (alternating sets of two different workouts with no rest between them) and peripheral heart action (moving from one workout to another without a rest, but alternating between upper- and lower-body exercises) and some light-resistance postural-enhancement work (exercises focused on improving and correcting posture).

'These specific resistance sessions form three to four workouts in Ellie's week, with room remaining to throw in some circuit-training sessions and anything else for fun!'

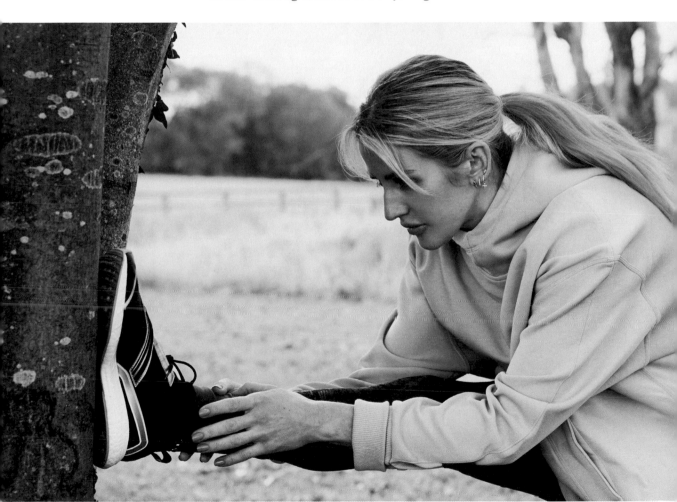

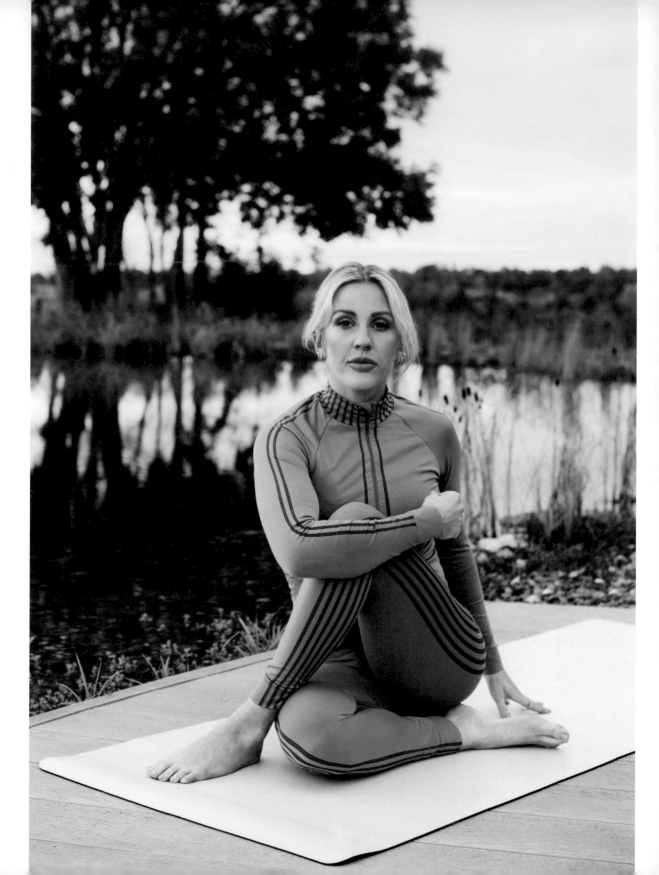

MATT ROBERTS' HOME WORKOUTS

'I've adapted the training I do with Ellie to create five workouts you can do at home, or in the park, or with no equipment. As I've said already, no two people are the same and we all have different moments of high or low energy, so think about what works with your routine and use the following as a framework for your training. You don't have to do the morning circuit first thing, for example, or the lunchtime circuit in the middle of the day. Life is busy; it's not always predictable. Do what works for you. And don't forget to warm up and cool down before and after each session.'

10-MINUTE AMRAP* – EARLY MORNING WORKOUT

This a great routine for fitting fitness into a busy day. It gives the whole body a workout. It can be done anywhere without any equipment.

Complete as many rounds of the below exercises as possible in 10 minutes.

Exercise	Sets	Reps or Time	Target Area
ROUND 1 (repeat)			
SQUAT	1	10	quads and glutes
PRESS-UP	1	10	triceps and chest
PLANK TO SHOULDER TOUCH	1	10	abs, chest and shoulders
REVERSE LUNGE	1	10	adductors, glutes, quads and calves
SPRINT ON THE SPOT	1	10 seconds	cardio, calves and hip flexors

See detailed instructions for how to do each exercise on the next page.

* AMRAP stands for 'as many repetitions (or rounds) as possible'

ROUND 1

SQUAT / 10 reps

How to do it:

- Stand with your feet shoulder-width apart or a little wider and point your toes slightly outwards. Contract and engage your stomach muscles.
- Keeping your heels on the floor and your weight back on your heels, lower yourself until your thighs are parallel to the floor.
- Go as low as you can while maintaining a straight back and ears over shoulders.
- Slowly return to a standing position by pushing up through your heels.
- And repeat.

PRESS-UP / 10 reps

How to do it:

- Place your hands on the floor just wider than shoulder-width apart. Keep your legs straight with your weight distributed evenly through your hands and toes. Keep your ears, shoulders and hips in a straight line.
- Contract and engage your stomach muscles then, keeping alignment, lower yourself until your nose almost touches the ground.
- Push through your arms to push back up to the starting position.
- And repeat.

PLANK TO SHOULDER TOUCH / 10 reps

How to do it:

- Start in a press-up position as above, with arms directly beneath your shoulders and your feet slightly apart and in line with your hips. Ensure your ears, shoulders and hips are all in a straight line.

- Keeping your hips still, lift one hand to touch the opposite shoulder.

- Now repeat on the other side with the other hand. This counts as one rep.

- And repeat.

REVERSE LUNGE / 10 reps

How to do it:

- Stand up straight with your feet facing forwards. Your feet should be hip-width apart.

- Step backwards one and a half stride lengths with your left foot, landing on the ball of your feet with your heel up. Maintain the position of your right foot. Both knees should now be bent at right angles and your back knee should not touch the floor.

- Push through the front foot to return to the standing position.

- Perform 10 reps, then repeat on the other foot.

SPRINT ON THE SPOT / For 10 seconds

How to do it:

- Stand with your feet hip-width apart and your arms by your sides. Hold a strong posture with your back straight and your head up.

- Start to run on the spot and increase to a sprint. Engage your stomach muscles, raise your knees towards your chest and pump your arms.

- Continue for 10 seconds.

NOW REPEAT THE WHOLE ROUTINE AGAIN FROM THE BEGINNING, AND COMPLETE AS MANY ROUNDS AS YOU CAN IN 10 MINUTES.

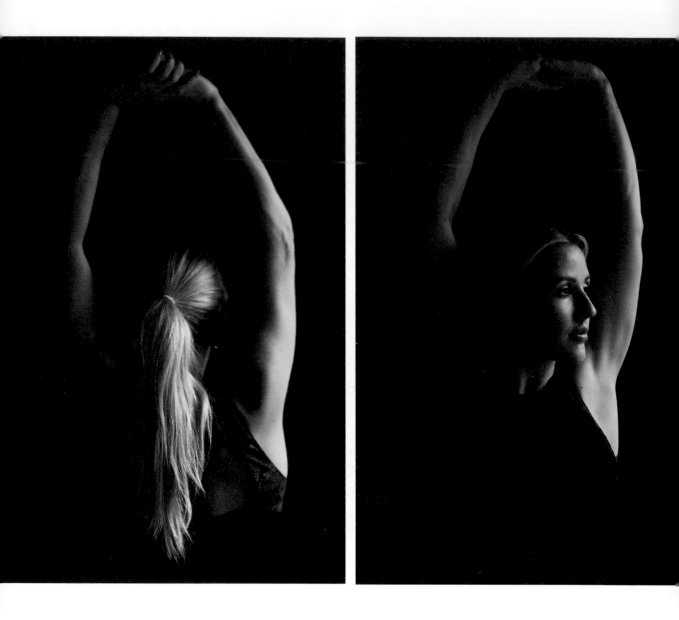

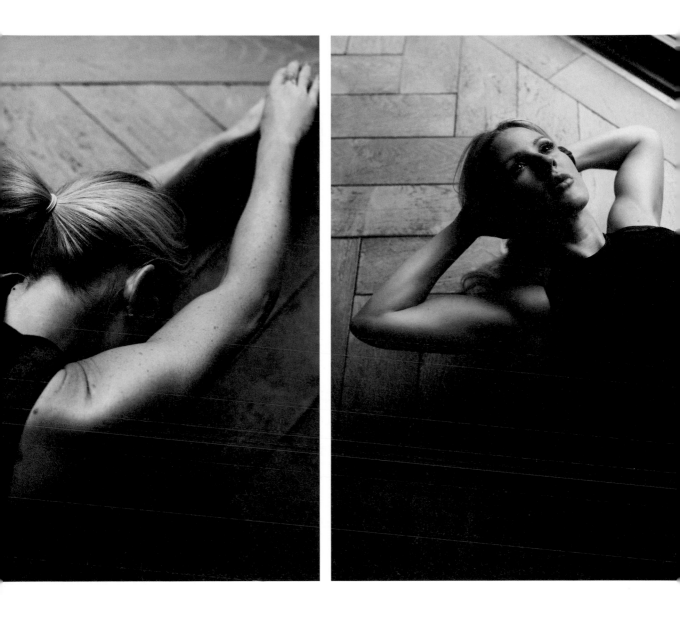

20-MINUTE LUNCHTIME WORKOUT

'This is a brilliant workout to do in the middle of the day – ideal if you're working from home as it will still leave you enough time to have some lunch and be back at work within an hour. If you're working in an office, or you're doing this at the weekend, just find a quiet room or some outside space to do it in. Like the routine on the previous pages, you don't need any equipment.'

There are 12 different exercises, each with 3 sets. It's split into 3 rounds with 30 seconds rest when indicated.

Exercise	Sets	Reps or Time	Target Area
ROUND 1			
PRESS-UP	3	30 seconds	triceps and chest
SQUAT	3	30 seconds	quads and glutes
BUTTERFLY SIT-UP	3	30 seconds	abs
MOUNTAIN CLIMBER	3	30 seconds	core, abs and hip flexors
30 SECONDS REST			
ROUND 2			
WALK OUT	3	30 seconds	core, abs, chest and shoulders
GLUTE BRIDGE	3	30 seconds	glutes
HOLLOW HOLD	3	30 seconds	core and abs
HIGH KNEES	3	30 seconds	abs and hip flexors
30 SECONDS REST			
ROUND 3			
PLANK TO SHOULDER TOUCH	3	30 seconds	abs, chest and shoulders
REVERSE LUNGE	3	30 seconds	adductors, glutes, quads and calves
AB BICYCLE	3	30 seconds	abs, core and hip flexors
JUMP SQUAT	3	30 seconds	quads, glutes, adductors and calves

ROUND 1

PRESS-UP / 3 sets of 30 seconds

How to do it:

- Place your hands on the floor just wider than shoulder-width apart. Keep your legs straight with your weight distributed evenly through your hands and toes. Keep your ears, shoulders and hips in a straight line.
- Contract and engage your stomach muscles then, keeping alignment, lower yourself until your nose almost touches the ground.
- Push through your arms to push back up to the starting position.
- And repeat.

SQUAT / 3 sets of 30 seconds

How to do it:

- Stand with your feet shoulder-width apart or a little wider and point your toes slightly outwards. Contract and engage your stomach muscles.
- Keeping your heels on the floor and your weight back on your heels, lower yourself until your thighs are parallel to the floor.
- Go as low as you can while maintaining a straight back and ears over shoulders.
- Slowly return to a standing position by pushing up through your heels.
- And repeat.

BUTTERFLY SIT-UP / 3 sets of 30 seconds

How to do it:

- Sit on the ground and bring the soles of your feet together. Let your knees fall open into a butterfly stretch. Pull your heels in towards your body.
- Maintaining this position, lie back onto the ground. Engage your core.

- Now sit back up with your hands loosely on the sides of your head. Roll your back up so that your lower back stays connected to the ground for as long as possible. Keep your feet on the ground at all times.

- Then roll back down to the ground again and repeat.

MOUNTAIN CLIMBER / 3 sets of 30 seconds

How to do it:

- Start in a press-up position (see page 181) with your arms directly beneath your shoulders and your feet slightly apart (in line with your hips). Ensure your ears, shoulders and hips are all in alignment.

- Engage your core and bring one knee towards your chest, then return it to the starting position.

- Repeat with the opposite leg and continue to alternate for 30 seconds.

30 SECONDS REST

ROUND 2

WALK OUT / 3 sets of 30 seconds

How to do it:

- Stand up straight with your feet hip-width apart.
- Bend at your waist and bring your hands to the floor.
- Keeping your legs straight and feet planted, walk your hands forwards until your body is parallel to the floor.
- Walk your body back in a bent-over position with your hands so that you are in the starting position.
- And repeat.

GLUTE BRIDGE / 3 sets of 30 seconds

How to do it:

- Lie on your back with your arms by your sides, palms down on the ground and knees bent with your feet flat on the ground.
- Slowly lift your hips off the ground until your knees, hips and shoulders are in alignment. Engage your glutes and abs.
- Hold this position for a couple of seconds, then return to the floor in a controlled manner.
- And repeat.

HOLLOW HOLD / 3 sets of 30 seconds

How to do it:

- Lie flat on your back and contract your abs as if to pull your belly button to the floor.
- Extend your arms and legs straight out with your hands and toes pointed.
- Slowly raise your shoulders and legs off the ground. Raise your arms and head in line with your shoulders. Keep your lower back in contact with the floor.

- Try to find the lowest position that you can hold without your arms and legs touching the floor.
- And repeat.

HIGH KNEES / 3 sets of 30 seconds

How to do it:

- Stand up straight with your feet hip-width apart.
- Maintaining a straight back, with your head up, lift your right knee while raising your left arm, bent in a 'running' position.
- Switch quickly, so that your left knee begins to lift before your right foot returns to the floor.
- Continue to alternate knee raises for 30 seconds.

30 SECONDS REST

ROUND 3

PLANK TO SHOULDER TOUCH / 3 sets of 30 seconds

How to do it:

- Start in a press-up position, with arms directly beneath your shoulders and your feet slightly apart and in line with your hips. Ensure your ears, shoulders and hips are all in a straight line.
- Keeping your hips still, lift one hand to touch the opposite shoulder.
- Now repeat on the other side with the other hand. This counts as one rep.
- And repeat.

REVERSE LUNGE / 3 sets of 30 seconds

How to do it:

- Stand up straight with your feet facing forwards. Your feet should be hip-width apart.
- Step backwards one and a half stride lengths with your left foot, landing on the ball of your feet with your heel up. Maintain the position of your right foot. Both knees should now be bent at right angles and your back knee should not touch the floor.
- Push through the front foot to return to the standing position.
- Perform reps for 15 seconds, then repeat on the other foot.

AB BICYCLE / 3 sets of 30 seconds

How to do it:

- Lie on the ground with your lower back pressed into the floor and your head and shoulders raised slightly off the floor. Place your hands loosely on the sides of your head.
- Lift one leg slightly off the ground and extend it out.
- Then lift the other leg, bending the knee and bringing it towards your chest. As you do,

twist through your core so that the opposite elbow comes to meet the raised knee. Don't move your elbow – all the movement should come from your core.

- Lower your leg and arm and, at the same time, begin to perform the same movement with the opposite limbs.

- Keep alternating for 30 seconds.

JUMP SQUAT / 3 sets of 30 seconds

How to do it:

- Stand up with your feet hip-width apart.

- Start to perform a normal squat (see page 181). At the point when your hips sink just below your knees, spring up through your heels and jump as high as you can.

- Allow your knees to bend when you land, immediately dropping back into a squat.

- And repeat.

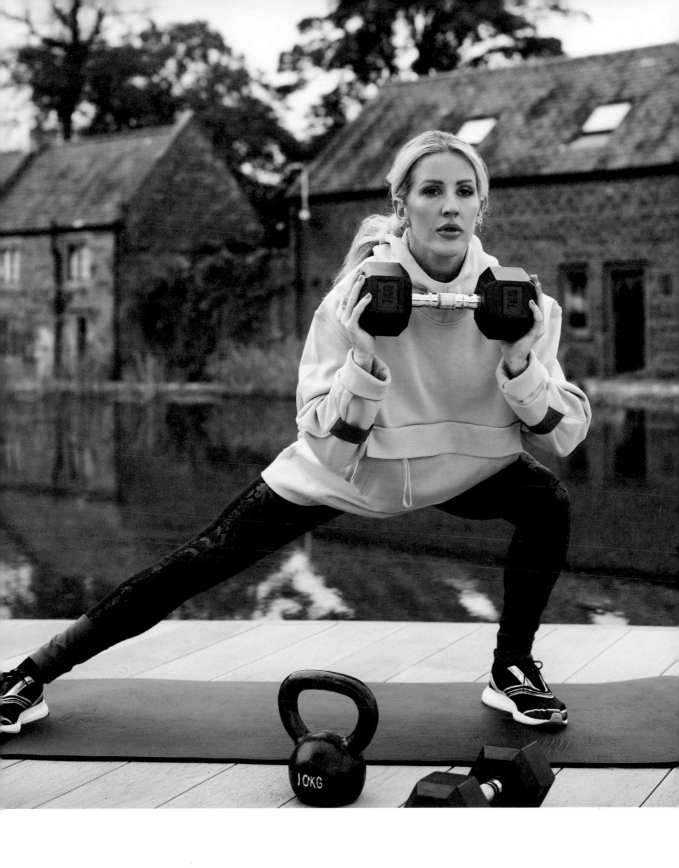

40-MINUTE AFTER-WORK WORKOUT

'This is a really good all-round body workout for when you have a little bit more time on your hands. You'll need a kettlebell or a pair of dumbbells (or household objects of similar weight, such as a tin of food or bottle of water), a large exercise ball or incline bench and a small box or step. There are 10 different exercises. It's split into 5 rounds with 45 seconds rest when indicated.'

Exercise	Sets	Reps or Time	Target Area
ROUND 1			
SPLIT SQUAT	1	20	adductors and glutes
ECCENTRIC PRESS-UP	1	20	triceps, pecs and shoulders
45 SECONDS REST			
ROUND 2			
SINGLE LEG DEADLIFT	1	20	hamstrings and glutes
SQUAT	1	20	quads and glutes
45 SECONDS REST			
ROUND 3			
LATERAL LUNGE	1	15	quads, adductors and glutes
W Y RAISE	1	15	shoulders
45 SECONDS REST			
ROUND 4			
SINGLE LEG STEP UP	1	20	quads and adductors
HIP THRUST	1	30	core and glutes
45 SECONDS REST			
ROUND 5			
SINGLE LEG GLUTE BRIDGE	1	15	glutes
TRICEP DIP	1	20	triceps and chest

ROUND 1

SPLIT SQUAT / 20 reps

How to do it:

- Stand with your feet hip-width apart and your toes pointed forwards. Step one foot forwards, as if performing a lunge. The heel of your back foot should now be raised.
- Slowly lower your body until your back knee almost touches the floor. Engage your core and maintain a straight torso.
- Push back up and repeat on the same leg for one set. Then switch sides.

ECCENTRIC PRESS-UP / 20 reps

How to do it:

- Place your hands on the floor just wider than shoulder-width apart. Keep your legs straight with your weight distributed evenly through your hands and toes. Keep your ears, shoulders and hips in a straight line. Engage and contract your stomach muscles.
- Keeping alignment, lower yourself more slowly than with a usual press-up, until your nose almost touches the ground.
- Push back up to the starting position.
- And repeat.

45 SECONDS REST

ROUND 2

SINGLE LEG DEADLIFT / 20 reps

How to do it:

- Stand up straight with your feet hip-width apart and your toes pointed forwards. Hold a kettlebell, pair of dumbbells or something of a similar weight in your hands in front of you.

- Lean forwards from your hips, with your arms staying straight and moving towards the floor.

- Shift your weight onto one leg while extending the other leg straight behind you, until your body forms a 'T' shape.

- Keeping a slight bend in your standing leg, slowly bring the extended leg back to the standing position.

- Repeat on the opposite leg.

SQUAT / 20 reps

How to do it:

- Stand with your feet shoulder-width apart or a little wider and point your toes slightly outwards. Contract and engage your stomach muscles.

- Keeping your heels on the floor and your weight back on your heels, lower yourself until your thighs are parallel to the floor.

- Go as low as you can while maintaining a straight back and ears over shoulders.

- Slowly return to a standing position by pushing up through your heels.

- And repeat.

45 SECONDS REST

ROUND 3

LATERAL LUNGE / 15 reps

How to do it:

- Stand with your feet together and your hands clasped in front of your chest.
- Take a big step out to the left side. Lower into a lunge, pushing your hips back, keeping your right leg straight and bending your left knee to 90 degrees.
- Push back off the left foot and return to the starting position.
- Repeat on the other side.

W Y RAISE / 20 reps

How to do it:

- Lie chest-down on a large exercise ball or incline bench, looking down, with your feet on the floor. Allow your arms to hang down with your elbows bent to 90 degrees.
- Maintaining bent elbows, raise your arms to the side of your body as you squeeze your shoulder blades together.
- Continue to raise your arms until they are parallel to the ground and a 'W' shape is formed.
- Slowely lower your arms back to the starting position.
- For the 'Y' raise, stretch your arms straight out in front of your head forming a 'Y' shape.
- Now repeat, alternating between the 'W' raise and the 'Y' raise.

45 SECONDS REST

ROUND 4

SINGLE LEG STEP UP / 20 reps

How to do it:

- Place a small box or step in front of you. Then place your left foot on the step.
- Keeping your left foot on the step, engage your glutes and push up to bring your right foot up onto the step. Do this in a fluid motion, maintaining a straight back and good posture throughout.
- Return the right foot to the floor and repeat.
- Perform 10 reps and then switch sides.

HIP THRUST / 30 reps

How to do it:

- Sit on the floor with your back against an exercise bench or box (or a sofa of similar height) with your knees bent and feet flat on the floor, shoulder-width apart. Rest your shoulders and elbows on the bench.
- Push through your heels to raise your hips and bottom up from the floor. Continue to raise until your thighs are parallel to the floor.
- Squeeze your glutes at the top, then return to the starting position.
- And repeat.

45 SECONDS REST

ROUND 5

SINGLE LEG GLUTE BRIDGE / 15 reps

How to do it:

- Lie on your back with your arms by your sides, palms down on the ground and knees bent with your feet flat on the ground.

- Slowly lift your hips off the ground until your knees, hips and shoulders are in alignment. Engage your glutes and abs.

- Keeping your right foot on the ground, extend your left leg below the knee and lift your foot. Your left leg should be straight and your thighs in line with each other.

- Hold this position for a couple of seconds, then return your foot to the floor, followed by your hips to the floor, in a controlled manner.

- Repeat, raising your opposite leg.

TRICEP DIP / 20 reps

How to do it:

- Sit on the edge of a chair or bench. Grip the edge next to your hips with your fingers pointing down.

- Press your palms down into the chair or bench and shift your bottom forwards off the edge. Keep looking ahead and keep your back and head straight.

- Slowly lower yourself until your elbows are bent between 45 and 90 degrees.

- Push yourself back up to the starting position and repeat.

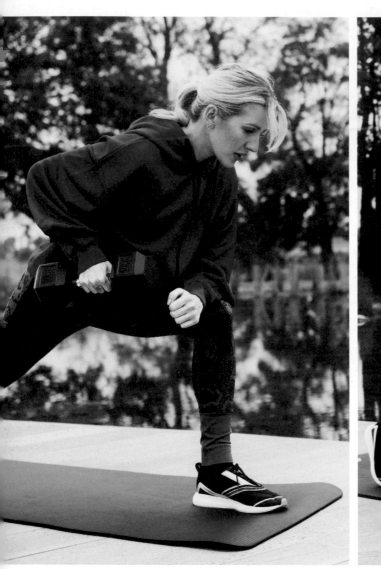
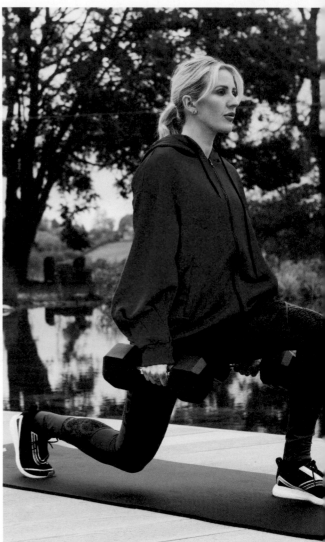

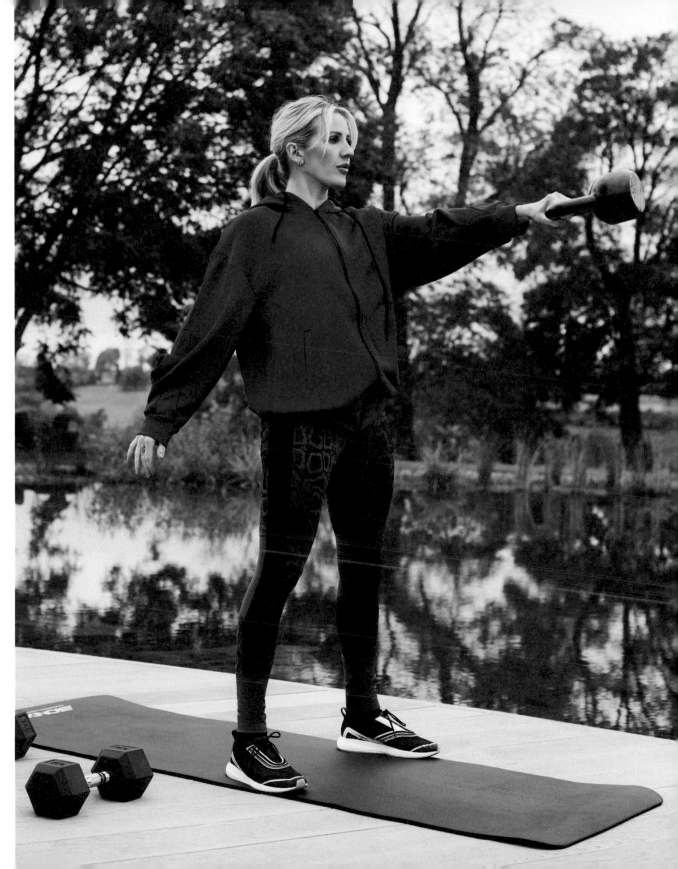

50-MINUTE FULL-BODY WEEKEND WORKOUT

'This is an all-round, full-body workout – great for when you have a bit more time and are looking to really feel the burn. This one is intense! You can do this at home or outside and will need a skipping rope and kettlebell (or something of similar shape/weight).'

There are 10 different exercises and 6 skipping sessions. It's split into 5 rounds with 30 seconds rest when indicated.

Exercise	Sets	Reps or Time	Target Area
SKIP	1	2 minutes	cardio
ROUND 1			
SQUAT	4	10 (hold 5 seconds each time)	quads and glutes
SINGLE LEG DEADLIFT	4	15 (on each leg)	hamstrings and glutes
30 SECONDS REST			
SKIP	1	200 skips	cardio
ROUND 2			
PRESS-UP OR HALF PRESS-UP	4	Until failure (i.e. you can do no more)	triceps and chest
REVERSE FLY	4	20 (maximum exertion)	upper back
30 SECONDS REST			

Exercise	Sets	Reps or Time	Target Area
SKIP	1	200 skips	cardio
ROUND 3			
REVERSE LUNGE WITH ARM RAISE	4	20 (on each side)	quads, adductors, glutes and shoulders
DEAD LIFT WITH DUMBELLS	4	20	hamstrings and glutes
30 SECONDS REST			
SKIP	1	150 skips	cardio
ROUND 4			
SHOULDER PRESS	4	20	shoulders and triceps
TRICEP DIP	4	Until failure (i.e. you can do no more)	triceps and chest
TRICEP OVERHEAD LIFT	4	20	triceps
30 SECONDS REST			
SKIP	1	150 skips	cardio
ROUND 5			
JUMP SQUAT INTO WALK OUT	3	Until failure (i.e. you can do no more)	quads, adductors, glutes, core and cardio
30 SECONDS REST			
SKIP	1	150 skips	cardio

SKIP / 2 minutes

How to do it:

- Hold the skipping rope with one end in each hand with your arms outstretched and feet close together.

- Swing the rope above your head and jump, lifting both feet a couple of inches off the ground, as the rope circles around to your feet. Focus on keeping your knees soft as you land and your core engaged throughout.

- Go as fast as is comfortable, aiming to increase your speed with time.

ROUND 1

SQUAT / 4 sets of 10 reps (holding for 5 seconds each time)

How to do it:

- Stand with your feet shoulder-width apart or a little wider and point your toes slightly outwards. Contract and engage your stomach muscles.

- Keeping your heels on the floor and your weight back on your heels, lower yourself until your thighs are parallel to the floor.

- Go as low as you can while maintaining a straight back and ears over shoulders.

- Hold for 5 seconds.

- Slowly return to a standing position by pushing up through your heels.

- And repeat.

SINGLE LEG DEADLIFT / 4 sets of 15 reps on each leg

How to do it:

- Stand up straight with your feet hip-width apart and your toes pointed forwards. Hold a kettlebell or something similar in your hands in front of you.

- Lean forwards from your hips, with your arms staying straight and moving towards the floor.

- Shift your weight onto one leg while extending the other leg straight behind you, until your body forms a 'T' shape.

- Keeping a slight bend in your standing leg, slowly bring the extended leg back to the standing position.

- Repeat on the opposite leg.

30 SECONDS REST

SKIP / 200 skips

ROUND 2

PRESS-UP OR HALF PRESS-UP / 4 sets, repeating until failure

How to do it:

- Place your hands on the floor just wider than shoulder-width apart. Keep your legs straight with your weight distributed evenly through your hands and toes. Keep your ears, shoulders and hips in a straight line.

- Contract and engage your stomach muscles then, keeping alignment, lower yourself until your nose almost touches the ground.

- Push through your arms to push back up to the starting position.

- And repeat.

- For a half press-up start in the same position, but only lower yourself halfway to the ground, contracting and engaging your stomach muscles and keeping alignment as above.

REVERSE FLY / 4 sets of 20 reps (maximum exertion)

How to do it:

- Stand with your feet shoulder-width apart holding a dumbbell (or a household object of similar weight) in each hand at your sides.

- Press your hips back in a hinge motion, bringing your chest forwards almost parallel to the floor. Allow the weights to hang straight down, with your palms facing each other. Maintain a tight core, straight back and keep a slight bend in your knee.

- Exhale and raise both arms out to your side, squeezing your shoulder blades together. Keep a soft bend in your elbows as you pull your shoulder blades towards the spine.

- Then inhale as you lower the weights back to the starting position.

- From start to finish, focus on proper breathing and the feeling of your shoulder blades coming together.

---

30 SECONDS REST

SKIP / 200 skips

ROUND 3

REVERSE LUNGE WITH ARM RAISE / 4 sets of 20 reps on each side

How to do it:

- Hold a pair of dumbbells (or a household object of a similar weight) at arm's length at your sides. Keep your chest tall and shoulders back.

- Step one foot back and bend both knees into a lunge position, while raising the weights in front of you to shoulder height, keeping your arms straight.

- Press through your front heel to return to the starting position.

- Then repeat on the other side. That's one rep.

DEAD LIFT WITH DUMBELLS / 4 sets of 20 reps

How to do it:

- Stand with your knees slightly bent, and your feet placed shoulder-width apart. Holding a dumbbell (or a household object of similar weight) in each hand with an overhand grip, so your palms are facing your body. Hold them in front of your legs.

- Bend at the hips and knees, lowering your torso until it's almost parallel with the floor. Let your arms hang down in front of your knees and shins. Make sure you keep your back in a neutral position, taking care not to round it.

- From this position, stand up straight without changing the shape of your back. Keep the weight in your heels.

- And repeat.

30 SECONDS REST

SKIP / 150 skips

ROUND 4

SHOULDER PRESS / 4 sets of 20 reps

How to do it:

- Hold a dumbbell (or a household object of similar weight) in each hand, with your hands by your shoulders, your palms facing forwards and your elbows out to the sides, bent at a 90-degree angle.
- Without leaning back, extend through your elbows to press the weights above your head.
- Then slowly return to the starting position.
- And repeat.

TRICEP DIP / 4 sets, repeating to failure

How to do it:

- Sit on the edge of a chair or bench. Grip the edge next to your hips with your fingers pointing down.
- Press your palms into the chair or bench and shift your bottom forwards off the edge. Keep looking ahead and keep your back and head straight.
- Slowly lower yourself until your elbows are bent between 45 and 90 degrees.
- Push yourself back up to the starting position and repeat.

TRICEP OVERHEAD LIFT / 4 sets of 20 reps

How to do it:

- Keeping your feet shoulder-width apart and your core tight, hold one dumbbell (or household object of similar weight) with both hands.
- Lift the dumbbell up over your head until your arms are fully extended with your palms facing the roof and your elbows pointing forwards.
- Bending the elbows and squeezing your triceps, slowly lower the dumbbell behind your head.
- And repeat.

30 SECONDS REST

SKIP / 150 skips

ROUND 5

JUMP SQUAT INTO WALK OUT / 3 sets, repeating to failure

How to do it:

- Stand with your feet shoulder-width apart and your knees slightly bent.
- Bend your knees and lower into a full squat position.
- Engage your core, propel your body up and off the floor, extending through your legs into a jump. With your legs fully extended, your feet will be a few inches off the floor.
- Land and control your landing by going through your foot (toes, ball, arches, heel).
- Stand up straight, then place your hands on the floor in front of you, just in front of your feet and walk your hands forwards on the floor, away from your body, until your body is parallel to the floor.
- Then 'walk' your hands back in, keeping your feet on the floor.
- Stand up straight, then jump into another squat and repeat.

30 SECONDS REST

SKIP / 150 skips

STRETCH ROUTINE

'This is brilliant at the end of a long day, or first thing in the morning, to stretch out your whole body. It's also great if you've been hunched over your laptop, sat down too long at your desk or slumped on the sofa, and will help to counteract the effects of sitting for a long time. For this routine you will need an exercise mat and may also want to use a foam roller or pillow for comfort.'

There are 10 different exercises, 3 sets of each. It's split into 5 rounds with 30 seconds rest when indicated.

Exercise	Sets	Reps or Time	Target Area
ROUND 1			
SIDE-LYING WINDMILL	3	10 (on each side)	lower back, obliques and QL (abs)
BIRD DOG	3	12 (on each side)	lower back
30 SECONDS REST			
ROUND 2			
CAT-COW	3	12	full spine
McGILL SIT-UP	3	10	abs and obliques
30 SECONDS REST			
ROUND 3			
THREAD THE NEEDLE	3	10 (on each side)	full spine and core
SIDE PLANK	3	30 seconds (on each side)	obliques
30 SECONDS REST			
ROUND 4			
90/90 HIP STRETCH	3	10 (on each side)	glutes
GLUTE BRIDGE	3	10 (on each side)	glutes
30 SECONDS REST			
ROUND 5			
SPIDERMAN	3	10 (on each side)	core
WALL SIT	3	40 seconds	quads

ROUND 1

SIDE-LYING WINDMILL / 3 sets of 10 on each side

How to do it:

- Lie on your left side with your left leg extended and your right leg bent across your body at a 90 degree angle. If you prefer, place a foam roller or pillow under your right knee.
- Keeping your left shoulder and hip on the ground, bring both of your arms straight out to your left side, placed on top of each other.
- Rotate your right arm up and over your head while trying to touch your fingers to the ground.
- Rotate fully around to the starting position.
- Pause briefly and then start again.

BIRD DOG / 3 sets of 12 on each side

How to do it:

- Begin on all fours with your knees hip-width apart and hands about shoulder-width apart. Draw in your abdominals.
- Lift one hand and the opposite knee an inch or two off the floor, while balancing on the other hand and knee, keeping your weight centred.
- Point your elevated arm out straight in front of you and extend the opposite leg out behind you. Your body will form a straight line from your hand to your foot. Keep your hips squared to the ground.
- Hold for a few seconds, keeping your back straight and your abs engaged throughout.
- Then return your hand and knee to the ground, and repeat on the other side.

30 SECONDS REST

ROUND 2

CAT-COW / 3 sets of 12

How to do it:

- Begin on all fours with your knees hip-width apart and hands about shoulder-width apart. Draw in your abdominals.

- Slowly lower your head, while you raise your back up, in the style of a cat arching its back.

- Then move into the opposite position, slowly raising your head and dropping your back into a downward arch.

- Then repeat, retuning to the 'cat' pose, with your head lowered and back arched.

- And then again into the 'cow' pose.

McGILL SIT-UP / 3 sets of 10

How to do it:

- Lie on your back on the floor, bending one leg while the other remains flat on the floor. Place your palms underneath the arch of your lower back.

- Slowly raise your chest, shoulders and head (together) off the floor, without bending your lower back. Imagine that your abdominal muscles are shortening and they are pulling your shoulders off the floor.

- Keep the position (you don't need to lift too far off the floor) for a few seconds, breathing deeply throughout.

- Then slowly return to the starting positon before repeating.

30 SECONDS REST

ROUND 3

THREAD THE NEEDLE / 3 sets of 10 each side

How to do it:

- Begin on all fours with your hands under your shoulders and your knees and shins hip-width apart. Keep your head in a neutral position and gaze down to the ground slightly.

- Breathe out, and slide your right arm underneath your left arm, with your palm facing upwards. Let your right shoulder come all the way down to the mat, resting your right ear and cheek on the mat and looking towards your left. Keep your left elbow lifted and your hips raised.

- Relax your lower back, breathe and hold for a few seconds.

- To release, press through your left hand and gently slide your right hand out.

- Repeat on the other side.

SIDE PLANK / 3 sets of 30 seconds each side

How to do it:

- Lie on your right side, with your legs extended out, propped up on the elbow of your right arm, which should be directly under your shoulder. Ensure your head is in line with your spine.

- Engage your abdominal muscles, drawing your navel in towards your spine, and lift your hips and knees off the floor while exhaling. Your body should be in a straight line with no sagging or drooping.

- Hold the position and keep breathing.

- Then as you inhale, return to the starting position.

- Change sides and repeat.

30 SECONDS REST

ROUND 4

90/90 HIP STRETCH / 3 sets of 10 on each side

How to do it:

- Sit on the floor on your sitting bones, with your feet on the floor in front of you, slightly wider than hip-width apart, and your knees at a 90-degree angle. Your arms should both be raised straight out in front of you.

- Twist your whole body to the left, keeping your hips and shoulders aligned, until your left knee and leg lie flat on the floor.

- Then twist in the opposite direction, keeping your hips and shoulders aligned, until your right knee and leg lie flat on the floor. It's like a windscreen wiper motion of your knees. Keep your arms raised up in front of you throughout.

- And then repeat.

GLUTE BRIDGE / 3 sets of 10 on each side

How to do it:

- Lie on your back with your arms by your sides, palms down on the ground and knees bent with your feet flat on the ground.

- Slowly lift your hips off the ground until your knees, hips and shoulders are in alignment. Engage your glutes and abs.

- Hold this position for a couple of seconds, then return to the floor in a controlled manner.

- And repeat.

30 SECONDS REST

ROUND 5

SPIDERMAN / 3 sets of 10 each side

How to do it:

- Begin in a standard push up position: hands on the floor just wider than shoulder-width apart. Legs straight with your weight distributed evenly through hands and toes. Keep your ears, shoulders and hips in a straight line.
- Drive your right knee up to your right shoulder and place your right foot outside of your right hand. Make sure your foot is flat on the ground.
- Slowly push your hips forward. Your left knee should touch the ground. Maintain this stretch for 10 seconds.
- Slowly pull your right leg back to return to the starting position and repeat on the other side.

WALL SIT / 3 sets of 40 seconds

How to do it:

- Lean back against a flat wall, with your feet shoulder-width apart.
- Pressing your back into the wall, slide down until your thighs are parallel with the ground in a sitting positon. Your knees should be above your ankles and bent at right angles.
- Keep your head, shoulders and upper back against the wall and hold the positon for 40 seconds.
- Push through your heels to return to the starting positon, take a short break and then repeat.

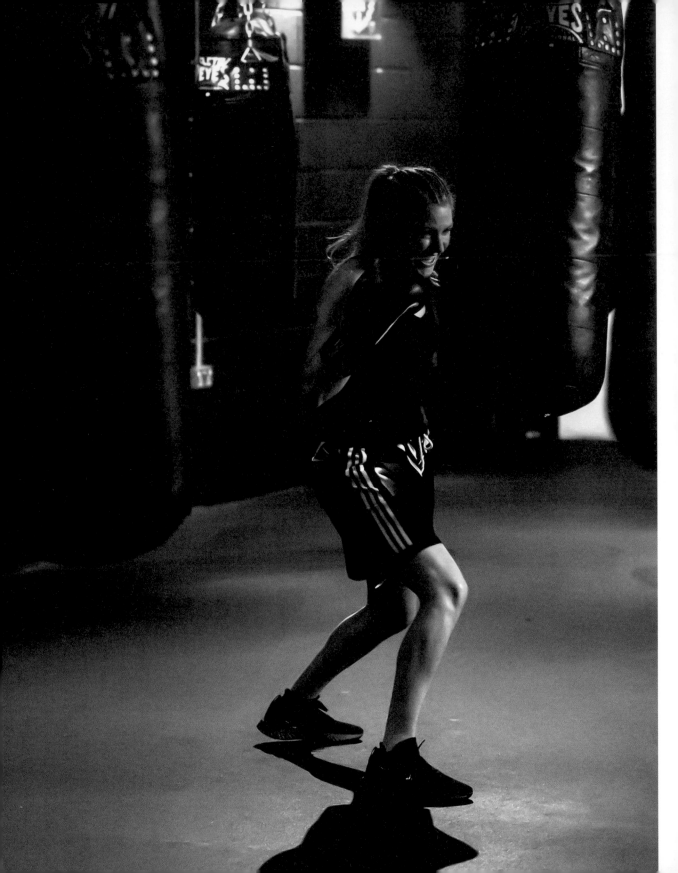

DARREN'S BOXING WORKOUT

'This is my dad's training regime from the 1980s and I still follow it to this day when I'm coaching.

'You should do three sets of the following ten exercises. Start with reps of six of each exercise, then eight of each, then finally for the last round do ten of each. If you're new to exercise, then you can cut these numbers in half and build up slowly over time.'

Exercise	Sets	Reps or Time	Target Area
ROUND 1		6 of all exercises	
BURPEE	1		arms, chest, core, glutes and legs
PRESS-UP	1		chest, shoulders, triceps, abs and serratus anterior
TRUNK CURL	1		abs
BURPEE JUMP	1		arms, chest, core, glutes, legs and calves
DORSAL RAISE	1		lower back, glutes and abs
TUCK JUMP	1		quads, glutes, hamstrings, hip flexors, calves, abs, biceps and shoulders
BOUNCE PRESS	1		chest, shoulders, triceps, abs and serratus anterior
SQUAT JUMP	1		quads, glutes, hamstrings, hip flexors, calves, abs, biceps and shoulders
SIT-UP	1		abs
PIKE JUMP	1		quads, glutes, hamstrings, hip flexors, calves, abs, biceps and shoulders
ROUND 2		8 of all exercises	
ROUND 3		10 of all exercises	

BURPEE

How to do it:

- Stand with your feet shoulder-width apart, keeping the weight in your heels and your arms at your sides.

- Push your hips back, bend your knees and lower your body into a squat position.

- Place your hands on the floor directly in front of you, palms-down, just inside your feet.

- Shift your weight onto your hands, then jump your feet back so you softly land on the balls of your feet, in a plank position. Your body should form a straight line from your head to your heels. Don't let your back bend at the hips or your bottom stick up in the air.

  (It's better to do this slowly and well, rather than quickly and with poor form, because then you won't work your core effectively. If you're a beginner, you can walk your feet back into the plank position, rather than jumping, until you get better.)

- Next, jump your feet back so they land just outside of your hands.

- Lift your arms overhead and jump up into the air. When you land, immediately lower into a squat for your next rep.

PRESS-UP

'This exercise can make a huge difference to your upper-body and core strength and works several muscle groups, including your shoulders, arms and core. If you're new to exercise, press-ups can be hard, but they're worth persevering with. The key is to learn how to do one properly, so they work all the right muscles without putting strain on your lower back.

'If you can't do a full press-up, drop to your knees, improve your form and then try to do them without your knees on the floor.'

How to do it:

- Start in a plank position, with your palms face-down on the floor, shoulder-width apart, and keeping your feet together. Look at the floor, but don't lower your head down. Engage your core as if you're trying to draw your belly button into your lower back.

- Bend your elbows back to a 45-degree angle and lower your body towards the floor, stopping when your chest is about elbow height.

- Breathe out and push into your palms to push your body away from the floor, returning to the starting position.

- Your entire body, from head to feet, should stay in a straight line throughout the entire move. Try not to let your hips drop towards the floor or rise up to the sky. Keep your neck neutral.

TRUNK CURL

How to do it:

- Lie on your back with your knees bent, feet flat on the floor, and place your hands on the tops of your thighs.

- Slowly lift your shoulders and upper back off the ground so your fingers slide up to touch your knees. Keep looking straight ahead the whole time.

- Slowly return to the starting position and repeat for the next rep.

BURPEE JUMP

'This is a harder version of a regular burpee and you'll need something to jump on that's low enough for you to feel comfortable. You could use a step (from the gym), a bench or a plyo box (you'll find these in most boxing gyms, regular gyms and you can buy them on Amazon). It needs to be stable and able to support your weight.'

How to do it:

- Stand in front of the box (or bench) in a squat position. Instead of dropping down to the floor to do a press-up, as you would with a regular burpee, place your hands on the box and do a press-up off it.

- Instead of jumping into the air, jump onto the box, keeping your feet hip-width apart and the weight in your heels.
- Land gently back on the floor, with your knees bent and your back straight, before repeating the exercise.

DORSAL RAISE

How to do it:

- Lie face down on the floor and place your hands next to your head so your fingertips are touching your ears (like you would during a standard sit-up).
- Slowly raise your chest off the floor about 4 inches and hold for 2–3 seconds.
- Slowly lower your chest back down to the floor and the starting position.
- Keep your feet on the floor during this exercise to avoid putting pressure on the lower back. Keep looking down at the floor, but don't tuck your chin under or move your head down.

TUCK JUMP

How to do it:

- Stand with your feet shoulder-width apart, lower yourself down into a squat position and then jump up into the air. Keep your back straight and tuck your knees up towards your chest as much as is comfortable.
- Land softly. You may need to pause before going into another tuck jump.
- Swinging your arms will help your momentum. As you get better at this move, you'll be able to jump higher and bring your knees closer to your chest. But if you're new to exercise, just spend time getting the move right to begin with.

BOUNCE PRESS

How to do it:

- Do a press-up (see pages 212–213), but on your way up, spring up and take your hands off the floor and do a quick clap, before landing on the floor again for the next rep.

SQUAT JUMP

How to do it:

- Stand with your feet hip-width apart and lower yourself down into a squat position.

- Keeping your back straight, eyes forward, press your feet down and jump off the floor as high as feels comfortable.

- Allow your knees to bend 45 degrees when you land, landing softly and keeping the weight in your heels, before lowering yourself back down into a squat again.

SIT-UP

How to do it:

- Lie down on your back, with your legs bent and feet firmly on the ground.

- Cross your hands to opposite shoulders or place them to the sides of your head. Don't 'pull' on your neck or head. Your core should be lifting you up.

- Curl your upper body up towards your knees. Exhale as you lift up.

- Slowly lower yourself back down to the starting position, inhaling as you lower your body back down.

PIKE JUMP

'The perfect pike jump is a jump where you bring your legs up in front of your body to form an L-shape, as you stretch out your arms to try and touch your toes. This is a cheerleading move originally, and it's a tough one, but a great all-over workout.'

How to do it:

- Start by practising with a simple jump up and down. If you have kids and a trampoline in your garden, it's a good place to practise.

- Swing your arms up and down again as you jump. As you jump, raise your legs upwards, so they're at a 90-degree angle to your body, trying to touch your toes as you do it.

- Keep your toes pointed during a pike jump. And keep your back straight as you land, with your knees softly bent, and land gently. Regularly practising touching your toes helps with this move.

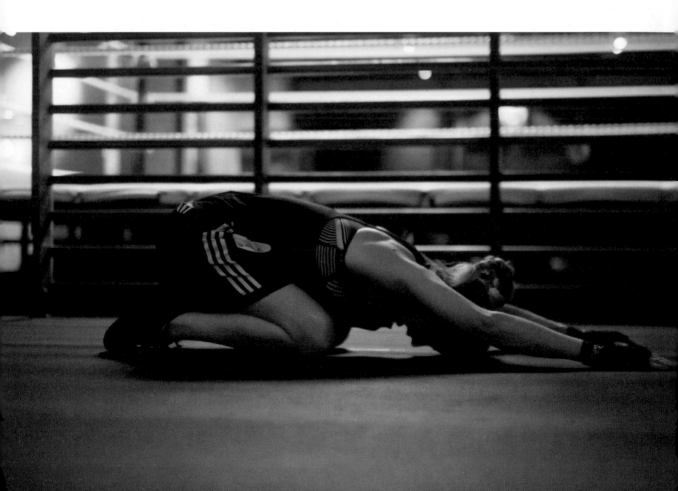

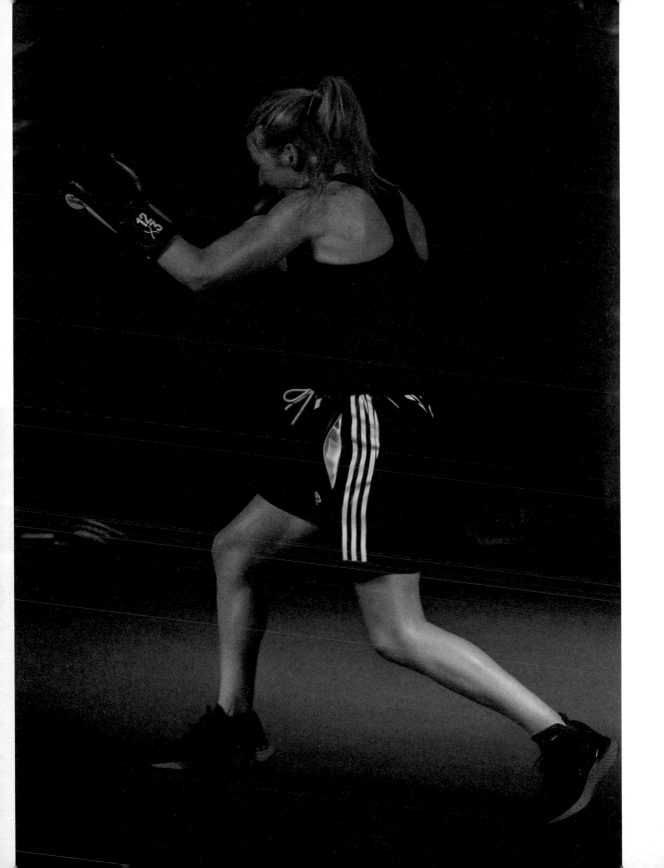

CATIE MILLER'S BARRE WORKOUT

'This is a home-based workout that you can do in your living room with very little equipment. When you start out I would suggest using a steady surface, such as a chair, a wall or a breakfast bar, to help keep you balanced. When you're ready, all these exercises can also be performed freestanding, although this will require more core strength and good balance.'

KEY TERMS:

First position: In the first position, your heels are together with your toes in a natural turn out with even weight distribution across all four corners of your feet. Never force the turn out. Bring your arms in front of your chest, palms facing in, arms gently bent at the elbow, as though you are holding a beach ball.

Second position: From first position, step your feet apart wider than your hips and shoulders with your toes in a natural turn out. Reach your arms out to the side, slightly in front of your shoulders. Maintain a soft bend of your elbows, keeping them rounded and lifted with your fingertips extended in an unbroken line.

Plié: This is the French for 'bent' and is used in ballet to describe the bend and stretch of your knees. *Pliés* may be shallow, so your heels remain in the first position (*demi-plié*) or deep, where your heels raise off the ground (*grand plié*). Remember in a *plié* you want your knees to wrap out over your 2nd and 3rd toes to ensure correct alignment.

Passé: This is the French for 'to pass' and is used to describe the movement when your working foot passes your supporting leg, bringing your toe to your knee.

Challenge zone: Your challenge zone or position is a place where you are able to dig a little deeper into your range, tempo or advanced options because you have grasped the technique effectively enough and can progress through the workout.

Exercise	Sets	Reps or Time	Target Area
HIGH KNEES	Up to 2	8	hamstrings, quads and lower abs
PLIÉ TO CURTSY LUNGE	1	8–16 (on each side)	hamstrings, quads and core
SECOND POSITION *PLIÉ*	2	8 (on each side)	quads
FIRST TO SECOND POSITION *PLIÉS*	1	8–16	quads and adductors
PASSÉ WITH LUNGE BACK	2	8 (on each side)	quads and hamstrings
TRICEP KICK BACKS	1	8–16	triceps with lower-body stabilisation
KNEELING SIDE LEG LIFT	1	8–16	abductors
PLANK	1	Hold for 8–16 counts	core and hip extensors
C-CURVE WITH OBLIQUE TWIST	1	8–16	core

HIGH KNEES / Up to 2 sets of 8 reps

Stand with feet hip-width apart and arms reached out in front of your shoulders in first position. Brush your right leg out in front of you, bringing your thigh and knee towards your chest. Keeping your back straight and arms strong, continue this movement, alternating leg lifts with a steady rhythm and pace.

Advancement: Work through the same exercise series with added weights (½–1 kg weights are great).

Cardio challenge! Add a light jog, bringing your knees up towards the chest as you run on the spot. Swing your arms in opposition, ensuring they are placed with purpose.

PLIÉ TO CURTSY LUNGE / 8–16 reps on each side

Stand with your legs open to a wide second position. Make sure your feet are naturally turned out and your arms are stretched out to the side from your shoulders. Cross your foot behind, keeping it in turn-out, bend both knees in each position and bring your arms to first. The working leg is moving as the supporting leg is anchored into the floor. Ensure your arms are moving from second to first as you transition into the movements.

Advancement: Continue for another 8–16 reps. Deepening your curtsy, hinge forward, reaching one arm long towards the floor as the other arm reaches in opposition above your head.

Cardio challenge! To finish, take your curtsy straight to a *passé* (toe to knee), adding a hop at the top before you place it back down into curtsy. Feel and embrace the hamstring and quadriceps burn!

Tip: Keep a proud chest, square shoulders and hips and even weight on front and back foot.

SECOND POSITION *PLIÉ* / 2 sets of 8 on each side

Standing centre or side-on to your chair, open your feet wider than your hips to second position with your arms stretched out to the side from your shoulders. *Plié* all the way down into second position, pressing through your feet and ensuring your knees are laterally rotated out from the hip. During the *plié*, focus on lifting your abdominals in and up. As you stretch your legs, press through your feet squeezing the backs of your legs (glutes and hamstrings) as you return to your starting position.

Advancement: Add a *relevé* (this is a classical ballet term that means 'raised': it describes the action when a dancer rises up and stands on their toes) at the top of the move to create instability and test your core.

Cardio challenge! Continue with the *plié* to *relevé* series, adding a jump at the top and softly landing through your feet into a deep *plié*.

Extra challenge: Try all three levels back to back to increase your heart rate. Try slowing it down or picking up the tempo!

FIRST TO SECOND POSITION *PLIÉS* / 8–16 reps

Carrying on from the second position *pliés*, alternating legs, step your outside foot back in to join your heels together in first position. Continue this action 8–16 times, working on stepping out to a wide second position with your toes turned out, knees wrapping back and your heels pressing into the floor.

Advancement: Once your rhythm and technique is set, you can advance by taking large jumps from first to second position. Focus on landing softly through your feet and keeping your chest proud. This will have your legs burning in no time!

PASSÉ WITH LUNGE BACK / 2 sets of 8 reps each side

Begin at an angle turned slightly in to your chair. Starting with your feet in first position, bring your outside leg to *passé* (toe to knee). *Plié* deep into your supporting leg, reaching your leg behind you towards the floor into a lunge as you hinge forward and reach your arm overhead. Straighten the supporting leg as you draw the working leg into *passé* and your arm back to first position.

Advancement: Add a *relevé* on your supporting leg as you bring the working leg into *passé*. Repeat for 2 sets of 8 on each side.

Cardio challenge! Continue the advancement series and add a hop at the top, landing softly through your working leg. Try all three levels back to back to increase your heart rate and work up that sweat!

Tip: Focus on maintaining a neutral spine, especially as you extend both arm and leg.

TRICEP KICK BACKS / 8–16 reps

Standing centre of the floor with your feet together, hinge forward from your hips and extend one leg behind you to a lunge. Ensure your weight is forward into your front leg and the back leg is straight with little weight placed on it. Square off your hips and shoulders. Reaching both arms behind, above your hips, with your palms facing each other or upwards, bend/extend the arms, keeping your elbows lifted. The bend is small. Concentrate on extending your arms to engage the triceps fully.

Advancement: Add a full range lunge driving your back knee towards the floor when you bend your arms and straighten your legs when you extend your arms.

Cardio challenge! Continue with the lunge/tricep kick-backs and add a lift of the back leg off the floor. Think about extending the leg longer, not higher, to activate your core and glutes for an added burn! Hold your leg and arms off the floor for your final balance!

Extra challenge: Try all three levels back to back to increase your heart rate. Try slowing it down or picking up the tempo!

KNEELING SIDE LEG LIFT / 8–16 reps

Begin in a side kneeling position with your hand placed directly under your shoulder and the opposite leg stretched out in line with your body to the side. Ensure your hips and shoulders are stacked and your knee is pointing forwards. Lift and lower your leg 8–16 times and then hold it up for a pulse.

Keep focus on your core, engaging it the entire time. Holding the leg in its challenge zone, slide it forwards and back, working the lower abdominals and glutes as it moves.

Advancement: Holding your leg to the side, flex the foot and continue to pulse your leg upwards. Reach the arm out in line with your working leg, and press it down as you pulse your leg upwards. This encourages the obliques to clench for an extra treat!

PLANK / Hold for 8–16 counts

Begin with your legs together in a plank position with your hands directly under your shoulders. Hold your plank for 8–16 counts.

Advancement: Continue holding your plank and add a *passé*, bringing the toe to your knee and your knee towards your chest to focus on core strength and lower abdominal connection. Alternate leg *passés* for 8–16 reps.

Cardio challenge! Continue alternating leg *passés* and pick up the tempo to a mountain-climbing run. Do 8–16 reps.

Tip: Remember to focus on your core strength. Lower down to your forearms if you have any wrist injuries. Keep abdominals in, chest proud and shoulders down. Think long neutral spine from the crown of your head to your heels.

C-CURVE WITH OBLIQUE TWIST / 8–16 reps

Begin seated, with hands placed behind your thighs. Tuck your tail under as you roll down into a c-curve position, ensuring both feet stay flat on the floor. Holding your challenge position, take small down-an-inch and up-an-inch movements – each time ensuring your tailbone tucks under, bringing your bottom ribs down to meet your hip bones.

Advancement: Continue this action while bringing your hands to first position. Hold your challenge zone and twist your upper body, alternating sides while creating a 'figure of eight' movement with your arms. Be sure to keep your knees and legs still.

To advance further, you can take the 'figure of eight' action over your head, challenging your upper abdominals.

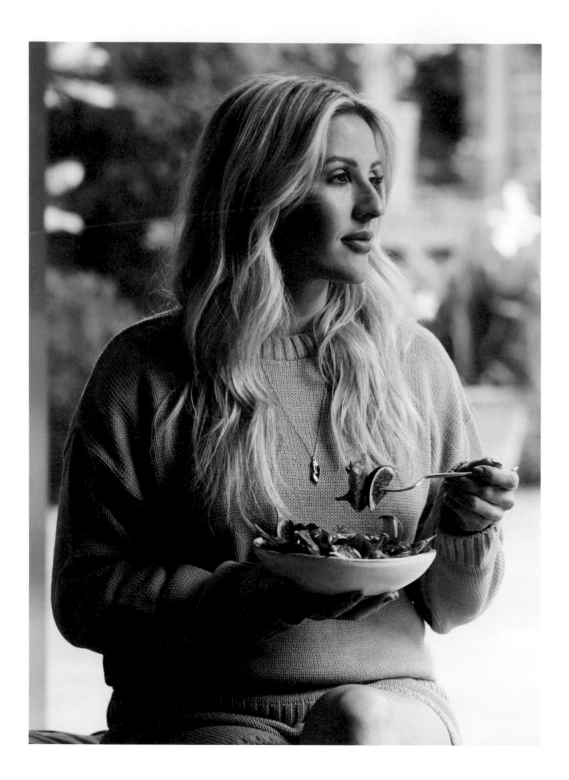

8

HOW I EAT: The Recipes

V Vegetarian

VN Vegan

GF Gluten-Free

DF Dairy-Free

BREAKFAST & BRUNCH

Smoothies

SERVES: each variation makes one large or two small glasses

Elsewhere in this book, I've mentioned my devotion to smoothies. This includes setting up a 'smoothie table' on tour to compete with crisps and snacks favoured by other members of the team. But now that I'm alert to my glucose levels I have a much more balanced approach to what I put in them.

But I do love whizzing up berries, greens and nuts for a quick and filling hit of energy to start my day. They are so easy to make. Simply blitz your choice of ingredients together in a blender until smooth. (Some blenders can't cope with too many nuts and seeds, but smoothies can always be poured through a sieve to make them extra smooth if preferred.)

Select your ingredients from the list opposite or on pages 230–231. I love to include blueberries in mine but try to choose a mixture of fruit if you can. When it comes to greens, I never use kale in smoothies as I find it too harsh, but make sure you pick something from this category as these are packed with nutrients. And I would only use herbs in a green juice, but that's a personal choice, so feel free to add some to any combination if you enjoy their flavour.

Some of my favourite combinations:

Energising Blueberry Boost

221 cals | 5.5g fat | 0.5g saturated fat | 6g protein | 9g fibre
32g carbs | 24g sugars | trace salt

150ml water

50g blueberries

50g cherries

1 orange

25g watercress

25g mint

1 tbsp chia seeds

1 tsp spirulina

¼ tsp ground cardamom

1 tsp honey

ice cubes

Revitalising Mango and Pineapple Blast

111 cals | 1g fat | 0.5g saturated fat | 2g protein | 4g fibre
22g carbs | 21.5g sugars | 0.5g salt

150ml coconut water

50g each mango, pineapple, carrot

25g spinach

1 tsp maca powder or lacuma powder

1 tbsp lime juice

¼ tsp ground cinnamon

1 tsp grated fresh ginger

ice cubes

CHOOSE YOUR BASE:

1 x 150ml
(or combination)

water

coconut water

plant-based milk

herbal tea

CHOOSE YOUR FRUIT AND VEGETABLES:

3 x 50g
(or a total of 150g)

any berries

plums

peaches

nectarines

melon

mango

pitted cherries

pears

kiwi fruit

seedless grapes

pineapple

papaya flesh

1 small peeled and deseeded orange/ satsuma/mandarin/ clementine

½ banana

beetroot

pomegranate

cucumber

avocado

carrots

PICK YOUR GREENS:

1 x 25g

spinach

lettuce

rocket

watercress

celery

wheatgrass

NEXT, THE HERBS:

to taste

mint

basil

parsley

lemon verbena

rosemary

fennel

1 lemongrass stalk

2 lime leaves

THEN THE POWDERS:

1 tsp

maca

cacao

baobab

lucuma

bee pollen

spirulina

ADD SEEDS/ NUTS/DRIED FRUITS:

1 tbsp

chia seeds

flax seeds

hemp seeds

sunflower seeds

pumpkin seeds

dates

goji berries

nuts

nut butters

FINALLY, CHOOSE YOUR EXTRAS:

FLAVOURS

¼ tsp

ground cinammon

ground ginger

ground cardamom

ground turmeric

vanilla extract

grated citrus zest

1 tsp grated ginger/ finely chopped chilli

1 tbsp citrus juice (lime, lemon, grapefruit)

SWEETENERS

1 tsp

honey

date syrup

maple syrup

coconut sugar

MAKE YOUR OWN SMOOTHIE

Grain-free Granola

MAKES about 8 portions

483 cals | 35g fat | 12g saturated fat | 13g protein | 6.5g fibre | 25g carbs | 19g sugars | 0.2g salt

75g coconut flakes, roughly chopped

50g dried bananas, roughly chopped (optional)

100g nuts – a mixture of any of the following: finely chopped brazil nuts or macadamia nuts, flaked almonds

225g seeds – a mixture of any of the following: pumpkin seeds, sunflower seeds, flax seeds, chia seeds

25g cacao nibs (optional)

½ tsp ground cinnamon

2 tbsp maple syrup

50ml coconut oil, melted

1 egg white, beaten (optional)

150g dried fruit – a mixture of any of the following: raisins, sultanas, dates, finely chopped figs, apricots or mango, pineapple, goldenberries, mulberries, cranberries, cherries, goji berries

This recipe will keep for a couple of weeks in an airtight container, so I often make a big batch of this and then have it on those days when I'm rushing out of the house early. There are no hard and fast rules about what to put in, so I've included some options below. I love the fact that you can get the crunchy, filling taste of granola without the grains, which can often leave me feeling bloated or uncomfortable.

Preheat the oven to 170°C and line a large baking tray with baking parchment.

Put the coconut flakes, bananas (if using), nuts, seeds, cacao nibs (if using) and cinnamon in a large bowl. Add the maple syrup to the melted coconut oil and pour this over the contents of the bowl. Mix thoroughly. If using the egg white, whisk this until frothy and add to the contents of the bowl – mix thoroughly again.

Spread the mixture over the lined baking tray, forming little clumps as you go. Bake for 20–25 minutes, turning halfway through and checking regularly to make sure it isn't catching.

Leave to cool, then stir in the dried fruit. Store in an airtight jar.

TIP: I've included egg white here because it really helps the granola stick together and crisp but isn't essential – the addition of flax seed helps, too, as it binds with the coconut oil and maple syrup.

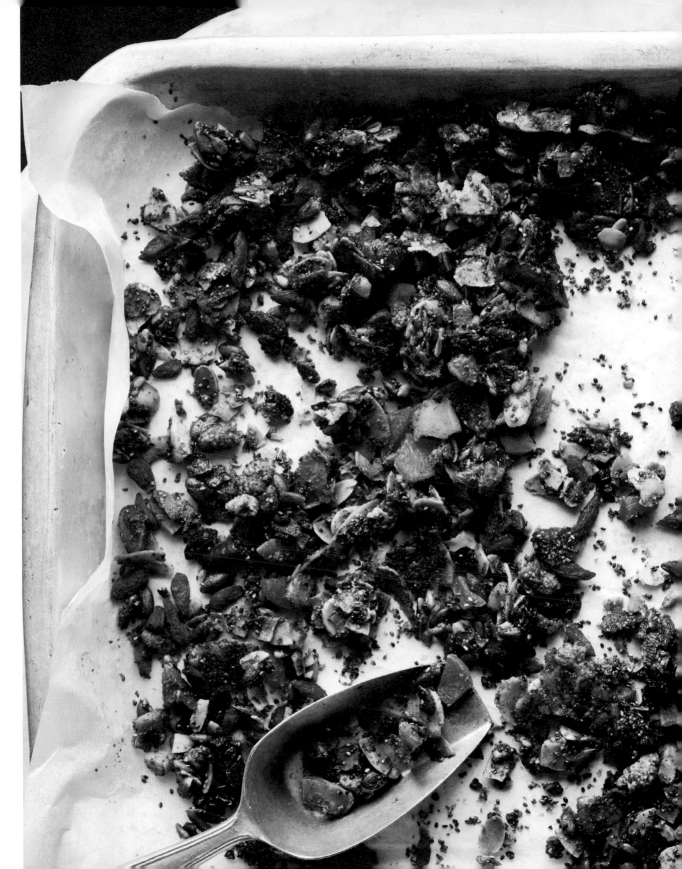

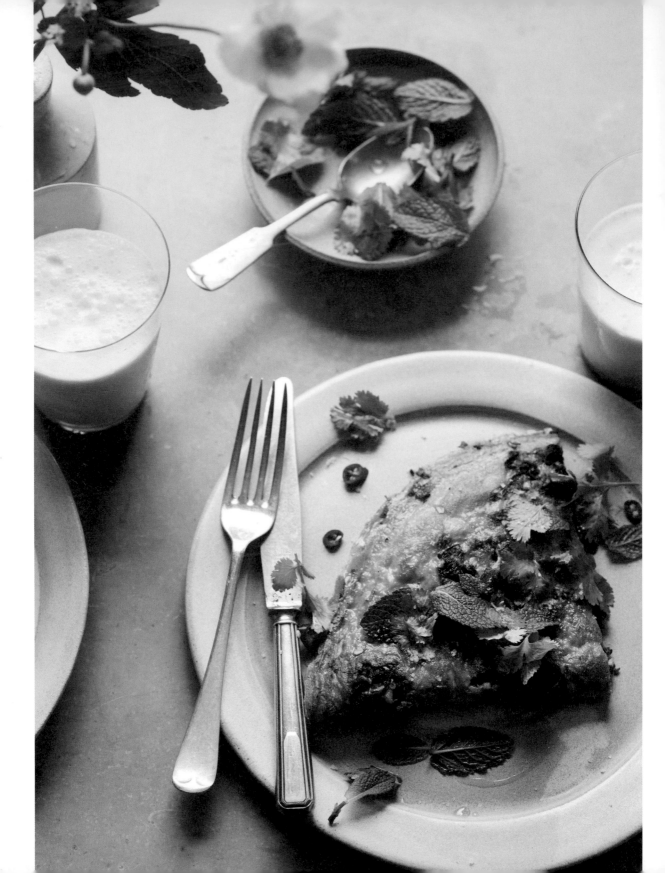

Masala Omelette & Lassi

SERVES 2

313 cals | 21g fat | 4.5g saturated fat | 23.5g protein | 4g fibre | 6g carbs | 5.5g sugars | 1.3g salt

100g spinach, fresh or frozen

1 tbsp olive oil

4 spring onions, finely sliced

1 garlic clove, finely chopped

15g piece of ginger, finely chopped

1 medium-hot chilli, finely chopped, plus extra to garnish, or 1 tsp hot sauce

2 tbsp coriander stems, reserving the leaves to garnish

¼ tsp ground turmeric

¼ tsp ground cinnamon

½ tsp ground cumin

4 eggs, beaten

salt and pepper

coriander and mint leaves, to garnish

For the salted lassi:

300ml unsweetened plant-based yogurt

2 ice cubes

a large pinch of salt

a large pinch of cumin seeds

This omelette is so easy to make and a great way to get some greens into your first meal of the day. I love spicy flavours, and this is one of my favourite weekend breakfasts – packed full of taste and goodness. The salty taste of the lassi is a great accompaniment.

If using fresh spinach, wash thoroughly and, while still wet, put into a small saucepan. Wilt on a medium heat until it has completely collapsed, then drain thoroughly. If using frozen spinach, defrost and drain, squeezing out any excess water.

Heat the olive oil in an omelette pan. Add the spring onions, garlic, ginger, chilli and coriander stems and cook for a few minutes until lightly coloured and aromatic. Stir in the spices and season with salt and pepper. Add the spinach to the pan, making sure it is evenly spread.

Season the eggs with salt and pepper. Pour into the pan and stir, pulling the egg in from the sides to the middle a few times and swirling to continually cover the base of the pan. Leave to cook on a gentle heat until just set – you want it still very soft in the middle – then sprinkle with coriander leaves. Fold over and cut in half. Garnish with the coriander, mint leaves and chilli.

To make the lassi, put the yogurt in a blender with 100ml water and the ice cubes. Add the salt and cumin. Blitz until smooth and aerated. Pour into two large glasses.

235

LIGHT MEALS & SNACKS

Socca – Gram Flour Pancakes

MAKES 2 large pancakes (SERVES 2 hungry people, 4 for a very light snack)

465 cals | 22g fat | 3g saturated fat | 19g protein | 11g fibre | 43g carbs | 3.5g sugars | 2.2g salt

150g chickpea (gram) flour

½ tsp dried mint

a pinch of ground turmeric

a pinch of ground cinnamon

2 tbsp olive oil

2 tbsp flat-leaf parsley, finely chopped, plus a handful of leaves to garnish

salt and pepper

For the dip:

25g capers

50g strongly flavoured olives, pitted and chopped

1 tbsp Dijon mustard

1 tbsp tomato purée

1 tsp red wine vinegar

zest of ½ lemon

½ tsp chilli flakes

a small bunch of flat-leaf parsley, finely chopped

When cooking these pancakes, the aim is to get them crisp and very slightly charred. You can either serve them on the table whole, to be broken off, with a dip on the side or cut into wedges a bit like tortilla chips. I love Mediterranean flavours, so I have also included a recipe here for a delicious tapenade that I think goes perfectly alongside. These are a real weekend winner for me – they taste even better after a Sunday-morning run.

Put the flour into a large bowl and season with salt and pepper. Add the dried mint and spices and whisk until the flour is lump free and everything is well combined. Gradually add 250ml water, whisking constantly, until you have a smooth batter.

Whisk in 1 tbsp of the olive oil and the parsley and leave to stand for at least an hour. You can also prepare in advance and leave to rest overnight if necessary.

When you are ready to fry the socca, preheat the grill to its highest setting. Heat a frying pan until it is too hot to hold your hand over for more than a few seconds. Brush half the remaining olive oil over the frying pan. Measure out half the batter and pour into the frying pan, swirling it to make sure it covers the entire base. When the underside of the batter has set and any liquid batter on top has thickened, transfer the pan to under the grill. When the top side of the pancake looks crisp and charred in places, it is done.

Keep the pancake warm while you repeat the process with the remaining batter.

To make the dip, put all the ingredients in a food processor or blender and pulse until you have a herb-flecked paste. Taste and adjust for seasoning, adding more salt, black pepper and vinegar as needed.

Sprinkle the pancakes with salt, more herbs, the dip and some whole capers.

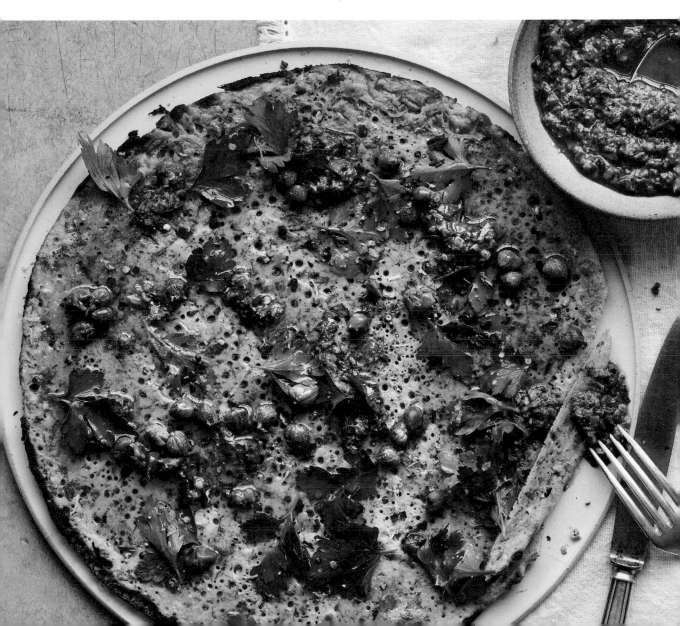

Tempura

SERVES 2 (generously as a light meal, 4 as a starter)

431 cals | 16g fat | 2g saturated fat | 8g protein | 4g fibre | 61.5g carbs | 14g sugars | 4g salt

For the batter:

50g brown rice flour

50g cornflour

½ tsp baking powder

1 egg yolk

80ml chilled sparkling water

salt

To fry:

1 litre oil (use light olive, rapeseed or rice-bran oil)

For the tempura:

a selection of vegetables (400g): sliced courgettes, carrots, squash, aubergine, sweet potato, whole or halved mushrooms, halved young artichokes, trimmed asparagus, trimmed spring onions, slim wedges of endives, small kale leaves, sliced sprouting broccoli slices of avocado, padrón peppers

a good combination would be: **100g asparagus tips; 1 small courgette or equivalent in other squash, sliced thinly; 6 trimmed spring onions; 2 Little Gem lettuces, cut into wedges**

Just about anything goes when it comes to what to tempura – the trick is to think about how dense things are and how long they are likely to take to cook when deciding how to cut them up. Hard vegetables like carrots are best sliced thinly, whereas asparagus can be left whole. It's a great way to use up leftover vegetables you have in the fridge. This is a really light batter – even lighter than a regular tempura as it is gluten free. It works really nicely with fish and seafood as well, especially prawns and calamari. For me, this is the perfect grab-and-chat food for when friends come round.

First prep all the vegetables and make sure they are dry.

Make the dipping sauce by mixing all the ingredients together. Taste and adjust to suit you.

Get everything ready for the batter. Put the flours, baking powder and a large pinch of salt in a bowl and whisk in the egg yolk. Have the water ready to add just before frying.

Get the oil ready by heating in a saucepan, wok or deep-fat fryer, making sure it isn't more than half-filled. When it is hot (it should be around 180°C), finish making the batter.

Whisk the water into the flour, keeping the mixing to a minimum – using a figure of eight motion with your whisk, just a couple of times should be enough. You want the batter slightly lumpy.

If you prefer a fish or seafood option: **use prawns; calamari slices; or white fish, cut into goujons (500g)**

For the dipping sauce:

3 tbsp soy sauce or tamari

2 tbsp mirin or similar rice wine

1 tbsp yuzu juice

1 tbsp clementine juice

1 tsp grated ginger

a pinch of chilli flakes

To serve:

a sprinkling of sesame seeds (optional)

Dip in the vegetables and fish or seafood a few at a time, gently shaking off any excess. Drop into the oil, being careful not to overcrowd the pan as this will make the temperature of the oil drop and could lead to soggy tempura. The tempura should immediately float. Cook until you can see the underside is turning a golden brown, then flip. When they are lightly but evenly coloured, remove with a slotted spoon and drain on kitchen paper.

Serve sprinkled with sesame seeds (if you like) and the dipping sauce alongside.

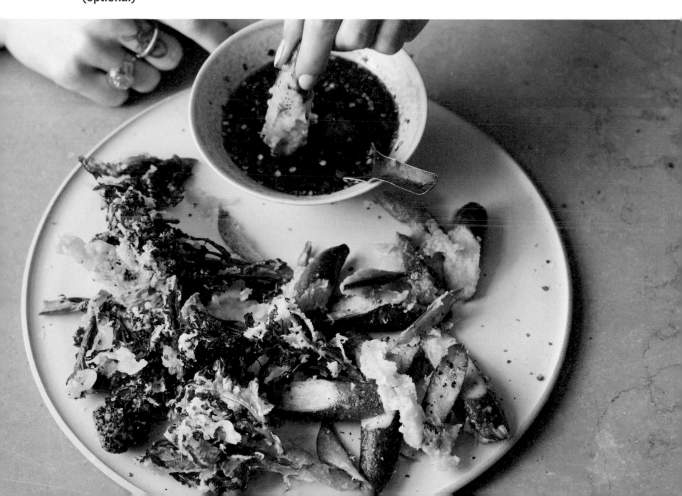

Harissa Grilled Sardines

SERVES 2

431 cals | 25g fat | 5g saturated fat | 43g protein | 4g fibre | 8g carbs | 7g sugars | 1.4g salt

For the sardines:

8 small sardines, filleted

1 tbsp harissa paste (below)

1 tbsp olive oil

For the harissa paste:

1 red pepper

4 red chillies

4 garlic cloves, left unpeeled

1 tsp cumin seeds

½ tsp coriander seeds

½ tsp caraway seeds

¼ tsp ground cinnamon

1 tbsp olive oil

zest and juice of ½ lemon

chilli flakes, to taste

This is a great lunch or light dinner. The saltiness of the sardines works beautifully with the mix of flavours in the grain-free tabbouleh. It would also be delicious with some seasoned, wilted greens. You can never have too many greens! This recipe also works really nicely with mackerel fillets. Use four fillets of mackerel for two people (rather than the eight sardines) – the cooking time will be around a minute longer.

I've included a recipe for the harissa paste, as I think this is the perfect accompaniment, but a shop-bought one can be substituted. You can also make a simpler version by just blitzing together some ready-roasted peppers, chillies and garlic.

First make the harissa paste. Heat a frying pan until it is too hot to hold your hand over. Add the red pepper and chillies, left whole, and the garlic cloves. Grill, turning regularly, until the skins of the chillies and pepper are blistering and blackening. Remove from the pan and put in a bowl. Cover with a plate and leave to steam and cool. Once cool enough to handle, remove most of the skin and seeds from the peppers and chillies and squeeze the flesh from the garlic.

Lightly toast the spices in a dry frying pan, then grind to a powder in a pestle and mortar or small food processor. Put all the paste ingredients into a food processor or blender and pulse until you have a thick red paste. Season with salt and pepper. Taste and add chilli flakes if you want it hotter.

Take the sardine fillets and slash the skin sides. Mix 1 tablespoon of the harissa paste with the olive oil and rub

For the tabbouleh:

small bunches of flat-leaf parsley and dill

1 small cooked beetroot, very finely diced

½ courgette, finely diced

½ red onion, finely diced

¼ cucumber, deseeded and finely diced

zest and juice of 1 lemon

½ tsp fresh or dried mint

1 tbsp olive oil

a sprinkling of sumac

salt

into the sardine fillets. Leave to marinate, covered, for at least 30 minutes.

To make the tabbouleh, chop the herbs as finely as you can, then mix with the vegetables, lemon zest and mint. Season with salt and pepper. Whisk the olive oil and lemon juice together and drizzle this over the vegetables just before serving. Sprinkle with the sumac.

To grill the sardines, heat a flat griddle pan or frying pan until it is too hot to hold your hand over. Wipe off any marinade from the sardines and brush with olive oil. Fry for 3–4 minutes until you can see that the skin is crisp and the flesh has just about cooked through, then flip over and cook for 30–60 seconds on the flesh side.

Serve with the tabbouleh and a squeeze of lemon juice.

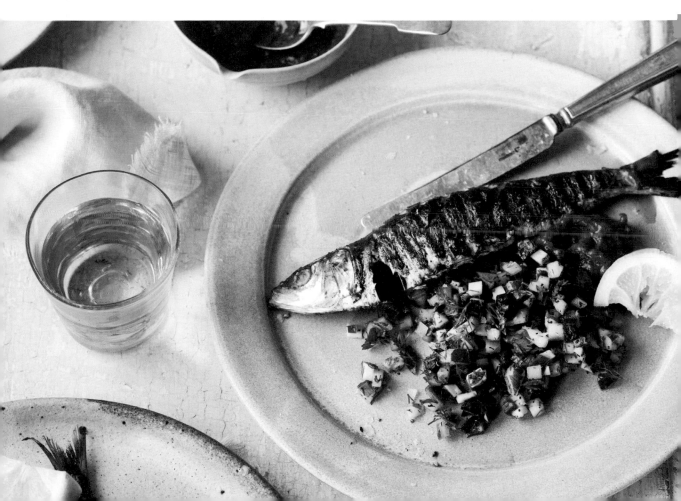

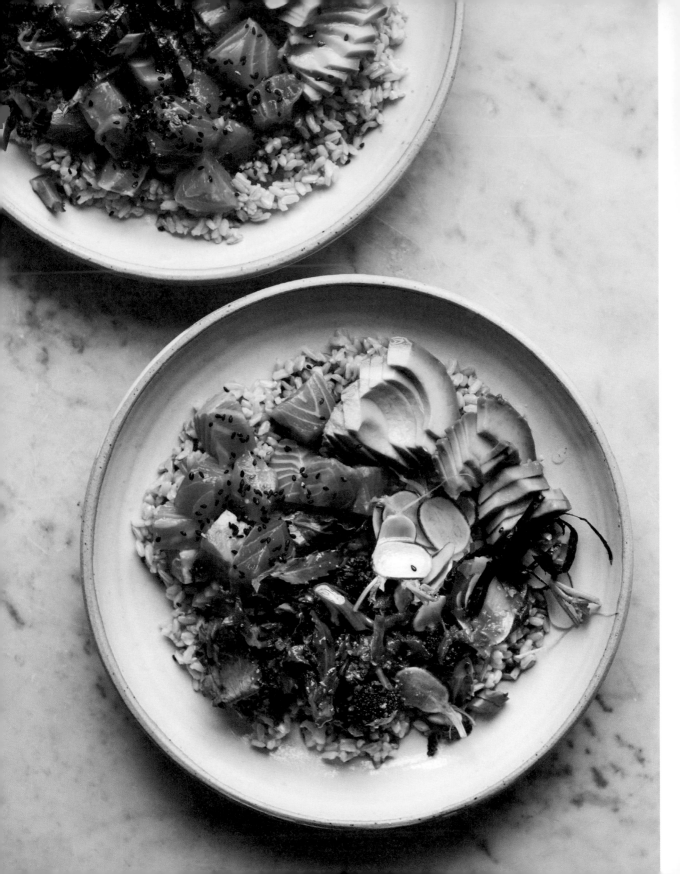

Poke Bowl GF DF

MAKES 2 BOWLS

489 cals | 27g fat | 5.5g saturated fat | 27g protein | 11g fibre | 28g carbs | 9g sugars | 2.7g salt

100g kale, shredded and blanched until tender, then well drained

150g sushi-grade fresh fish fillet, very well chilled

100g cooked brown rice

200g sprouting broccoli/ Tenderstem, blanched and thinly sliced

6 radishes, finely sliced

1 avocado, sliced

salt and pepper

For the dressing:

2 tbsp soy sauce or tamari

1 tbsp rice vinegar

1 tbsp mirin

1 tbsp yuzu or grapefruit juice

1 tsp sesame oil

1 tsp wasabi paste

a few pieces of sushi ginger, finely sliced

To serve:

small piece of nori, shredded (or 2 tbsp seaweed salad)

2 spring onions, finely chopped

a few snips of cress or other micro leaves

a sprinkling of black sesame seeds

dash of hot sauce (optional)

This delicious bowl is packed full of goodness and flavour – it's one of my favourite light meals. The protein from the fish is perfect if you're training and the fibre from the vegetables will keep you full for hours. Any fish can be used for this as long as it is sushi/sashimi grade and has been flash frozen. Oily fish tend to work best, but it's also good with a white fish such as sea bass or red fish. Or a vegan version can be made with diced silken tofu.

Make the dressing by whisking all the ingredients together and seasoning with salt.

To assemble the bowls, divide the kale between two bowls, season well with salt and pepper, then drizzle over a little of the dressing. Arrange the fish, brown rice, broccoli, radishes and avocado on top in separate piles and add more of the dressing. Garnish with the nori, spring onions, micro leaves and sesame seeds. Serve with a few dashes of hot sauce if you would like extra heat.

243

SALADS & SOUPS

Shrimp, Avocado & Quinoa Salad

SERVES 2

457 cals | 30g fat | 5.5g saturated fat | 17g protein | 7g fibre | 26g carbs | 10g sugars | 1.1g salt

For the shrimp:

1 jalapeño, roughly chopped

1 garlic clove

zest of 2 limes

1 tbsp olive oil

150g raw peeled shrimp
or prawns

salt and pepper

For the salad:

100g cooked quinoa (see
Tip) – a mixture of black, red
and white is good

75g baby spinach leaves

75g watercress sprigs

juice of 1 lime

1 avocado, peeled and sliced

½ small mango, peeled and
diced (optional)

4 spring onions, shredded

handful of coriander or mint
leaves (or both)

For the dressing:

1 tbsp olive oil

juice of 1 lime

1 tsp chipotle paste

¼ tsp honey

This is a lovely summer salad – lots of great colours, flavours and textures. The mango in this is optional (as I know fruit in salad is a bit Marmite), but it works really well with the heat and pepper of the chilli and watercress. You need to marinate the shrimp for at least an hour to get the best flavour, but it's totally worth it – and then it's really quick to pull it all together. It's fine to use ready-cooked quinoa if you prefer, but it's cheaper and tastier to cook your own!

First make the shrimp marinade. Put the jalapeño, garlic and lime zest into a small food processor or blender with the olive oil and plenty of salt and pepper. Pulse to a fine paste. Put the shrimp in a small bowl and cover with the marinade. Cover the bowl and leave for at least an hour.

To cook the shrimp, heat a griddle pan until hot. Brush off any excess marinade and grill the shrimp until pink, opaque and very lightly charred.

To assemble the salad, arrange the quinoa over two plates and top with the spinach and watercress. Put the lime juice in a bowl with a generous pinch of salt and drop in the avocado slices. Toss to coat with the lime juice, then add these to the salad, along with the diced mango, if using.

Whisk the dressing ingredients together and season with salt and pepper. Thin with a little water if too thick, then drizzle over the salad. Top with the shrimp, the spring onions and herbs.

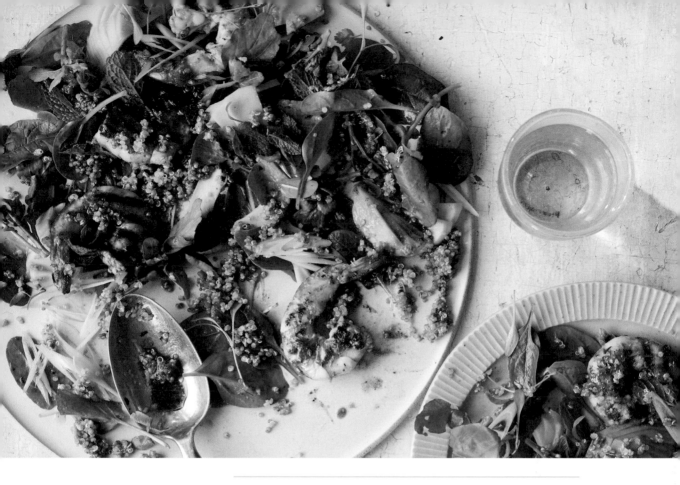

TIP: To cook 100g quinoa, put the quinoa in a sieve and run it under cold water for at least 30 seconds to remove the bitter outer coating. Transfer to a bowl of cold water and leave to soak for 5 minutes. Drain and put in a saucepan with 1 teaspoon coconut or olive oil. Fry until it is quite dry and smells nutty, then add 150ml water or vegetable stock. Season with salt and bring to the boil. Turn down the heat and cover. Cook for 12 minutes, then remove from the heat and leave covered for at least another 5 minutes – it will continue to steam in the residual heat. Fluff with a fork.

NOTE: Around 30g uncooked quinoa will give 100g cooked, but it seems odd to cook that amount as it's so small. However, it does keep well in the fridge for a week and can also be frozen.

Roast Red Cabbage Salad

SERVES 2

779 cals | 49g fat | 8g saturated fat | 36g protein | 16g fibre | 40g carbs | 16g sugars | 1.6g salt

½ small red cabbage, cut into slim wedges

2 small heads endive, cut into wedges

1 tbsp olive oil

75g bag of greens – beetroot greens and mustard greens are good

100g Puy lentils, cooked

1 pear, sliced into wedges

2 small smoked mackerel fillets, skinned and roughly torn (optional)

1 tbsp pumpkin seeds, or 2 tbsp walnuts, hazelnuts or pecans

leaves from a sprig of thyme

handful of flat-leaf parsley leaves

salt and pepper

For the dressing:

2 tbsp olive oil or nut oil (walnut or hazelnut)

2 tsp wholegrain mustard

½ tsp honey (optional)

1 tbsp sherry or red wine vinegar

1 tbsp orange juice

Red cabbage isn't just for roast dinners! I think it's a great vegetable – it's packed full of vitamin C, making it a brilliant immune booster, and also low in calories and fat, but high in fibre. You can eat it raw, sautéed, pickled, but I love the sweetness you get when it's roasted like this. The flavour combinations in this salad work so well with each other and it's easy to throw together, too.

Preheat the oven to 200ºC. Arrange the cabbage and endive in a roasting tin, making sure they have plenty of space around them. Drizzle with the olive oil and season with salt and pepper. Roast for 30–35 minutes, turning over once, until tender at the core and slightly crisp and brown around the edges. Leave to cool to room temperature.

Arrange the roasted cabbage and endive on two salad plates with the greens, lentils, sliced pear and mackerel fillets, if using.

Whisk all the ingredients for the dressing together and season with salt and pepper. Drizzle over the salad and garnish with the pumpkin seeds or nuts and herbs.

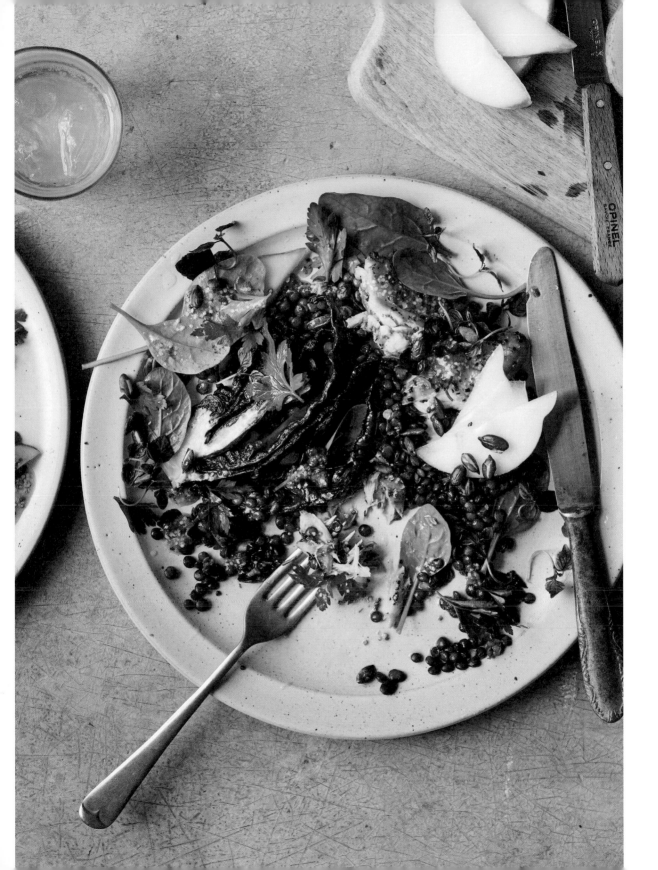

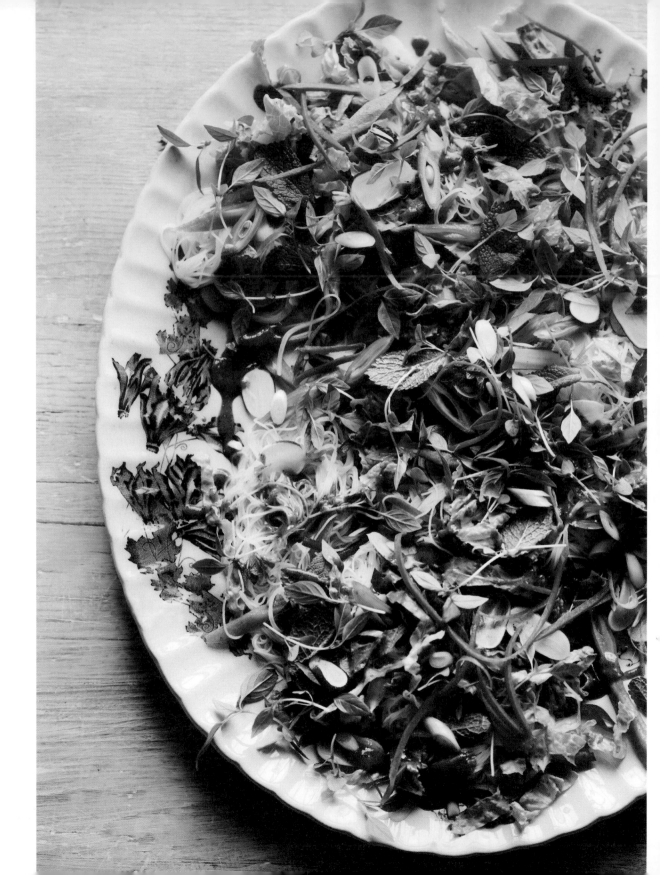

Glass Noodle Salad

SERVES 2

328 cals | 11g fat | 2g saturated fat | 12g protein | 8g fibre | 42g carbs | 14g sugars | 2.2g salt

75g dried glass noodles

1 carrot, julienned

½ red pepper, very finely sliced

100g runner or flat beans, trimmed and finely shredded

2 Little Gem lettuces, shredded

6 radishes, finely sliced

4 spring onions, finely sliced on the diagonal

small bunch of mint

small bunch of Thai basil

2 pitted dates, very finely chopped

1 tbsp pumpkin seeds

1 tsp black sesame seeds

For the dressing:

1 tbsp nut butter (any sort: peanut butter is traditional, or cashew nut would be good)

½ tsp honey or palm sugar

15g ginger, grated

1 garlic clove, crushed or grated

1 tbsp fish sauce or soy sauce

juice and zest of 1 lime

½ tsp hot sauce

½ tsp sesame oil

salt and pepper

This is another big favourite for me – I like to make it with glass noodles (either sweet potato or mung bean) but it works with any vermicelli or fine noodles. Cut the vegetables into long, thin strips, so they mirror and work alongside the noodles. It's a great dish to do when you have people over as you can just put a big bowl in the middle of the table and let everyone help themselves.

First cook the glass noodles according to the packet instructions. This will normally be a case of soaking them until pliable, then plunging them into boiling water for 2–3 minutes. The texture shouldn't be too soft – they should be slightly chewy. Run under cold water until cool, then drain thoroughly.

Put the noodles in a bowl with all the vegetables. Reserve a few small mint and basil leaves for a garnish and shred the rest. Add these to the salad and stir in the dates.

Make the dressing by whisking all the ingredients together until smooth. Season with salt and pepper. Pour the dressing over the salad and mix thoroughly. Divide between two bowls and sprinkle with the pumpkin seeds, sesame seeds and reserved herbs.

Lentil & Greens Soup

SERVES 4

315 cals | 8g fat | 1.5g saturated fat | 19g protein | 12g fibre | 37g carbs | 7.5g sugars | 0.7g salt

2 tbsp olive oil

1 large onion, finely chopped

1 stick celery, finely chopped

1 carrot, finely chopped (optional)

3 garlic cloves, crushed or grated

1 tsp dried thyme or 1 large sprig of thyme

1 tbsp tomato purée

250g brown lentils

1–1.5 litres vegetable stock

300g spinach (fresh or frozen), Swiss chard or any type of kale, shredded

juice of 1/2–1 lemon, according to taste

salt and pepper

To serve:

a few parsley or mint leaves, shredded

TIP: Herb garnish – flat-leaf parsley will enhance the savouriness of the soup; the mint lifts it and gives it a fresher edge. Use either or both.

Nothing beats a delicious, warming soup when you need a bit of a boost. This is a great rich savoury one and an all-round good blueprint recipe – if you want a bit more flavour, add some ginger and spices along with the garlic; if you fancy it more like a dal, just add a bit less water. It freezes well too, so I tend to cook a big batch at a time.

Heat the olive oil in a large saucepan or casserole. Add the onion, celery and carrot and sauté gently until soft and translucent. Add the garlic and thyme and cook for a further couple of minutes. Add the tomato purée and stir until it starts to separate and has a rich aroma.

Add the lentils and stir to coat, then pour in a litre of the stock. Season generously with salt and pepper (lentils like a lot of salt), then bring to the boil. Turn down the heat and partially cover, then leave to simmer until the lentils are tender – this will take up to 45 minutes.

Add the greens, pushing them into the liquid with a wooden spoon until they are all immersed, then cook until completely tender – this will take no time at all for the spinach, slightly longer for the chard or kale. Check liquid levels – add more stock at this stage if you think it needs it.

Taste and adjust the seasoning, then add plenty of lemon juice. Remove the thyme sprig if used, then leave it chunky if you like, or – and this is easier to eat – blitz very briefly with a stick blender so that the greens are broken up but the soup still has plenty of texture.

Serve with a sprinkling of parsley and/or mint.

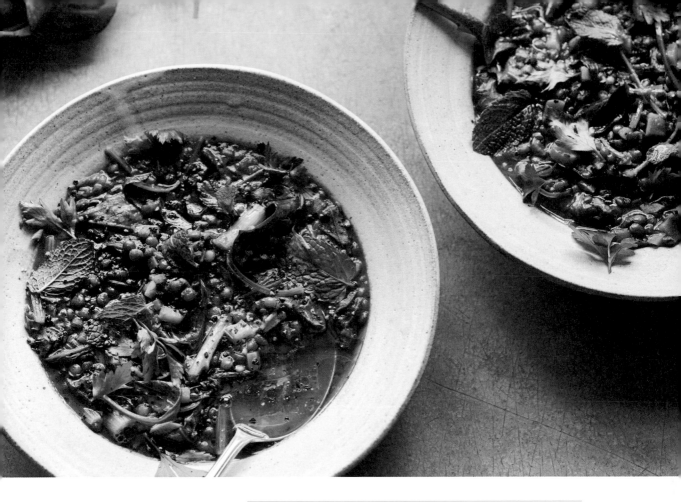

SPEED IT UP: Use red lentils instead, which will cook in 20 minutes. These will break down more than the brown, so will give the soup a smoother texture.

SPICE IT UP: Add 15g grated ginger and 2 tbsp coriander stems with the garlic, along with your favourite spice/curry mix OR 1 tsp ground turmeric, 1 tsp cayenne, 1 tsp ground cumin, 1 tsp ground coriander, ½ tsp ground cinnamon, ½ tsp ground cardamom. Garnish with coriander or mint in place of the parsley.

Fish Chowder GF DF

SERVES 2 generously

583 cals | 19g fat | 3g saturated fat | 70g protein | 15g fibre | 28g carbs | 15g sugars | 2.9g salt

2 tbsp olive oil

1 onion, diced

2 leeks, whites only, cut into rounds

150g cauliflower, cut into small pieces

150g celeriac, peeled and diced

2 garlic cloves, finely chopped

bouquet garni of 2 bay leaves and 2 sprigs of flat-leaf parsley

400ml fish or vegetable stock

200ml plant-based milk (e.g. soy)

200g sweetcorn (frozen is best)

250g white fish fillets (eg. cod or haddock), cut into chunks

250g smoked haddock, preferably undyed, cut into chunks

100g North Atlantic peeled prawns

small bunch of dill or chervil, fronds torn

salt and pepper

dash of Tabasco, to serve (optional)

This super-simple fish chowder is the perfect comfort food. For this healthy twist on a classic dish you can use pretty much any firm white fish you have. To make it really luxurious, replace 50ml of the plant-based milk with plant-based double cream – but add this at the end, at the same time as the prawns.

Heat the olive oil in a large saucepan or casserole. Add the onion, leeks, cauliflower, celeriac, garlic and the bouquet garni. Stir to coat with the oil and sauté very gently for 5 minutes, then add a splash of water, cover, and leave to braise until the vegetables are completely tender. Mash very lightly once or twice with the back of a wooden spoon, just to break up some of the cauliflower and celeriac.

Season with salt and pepper, then pour in the stock and milk. Add the sweetcorn. Bring almost to the boil, then, keeping the heat on low, add the white fish and smoked haddock. Allow it to poach very gently (if you do this on too high a heat, the fish will become tough) until it has turned opaque and just cooked through, then stir in the prawns and most of the herbs.

Remove the bouquet garni, then ladle into soup bowls. Serve with a garnish of dill or chervil and a dash of Tabasco for a little extra heat, if you like.

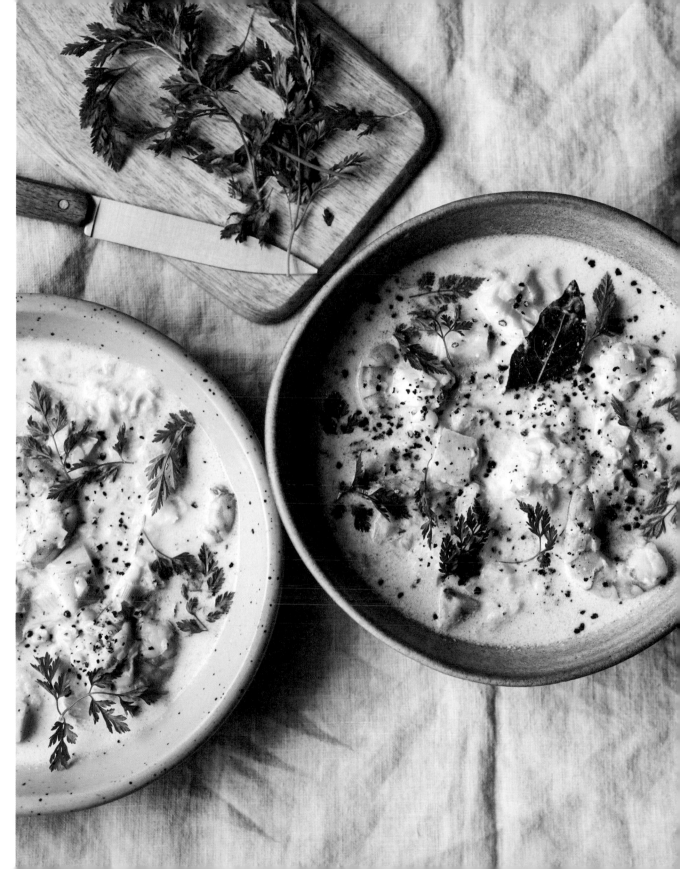

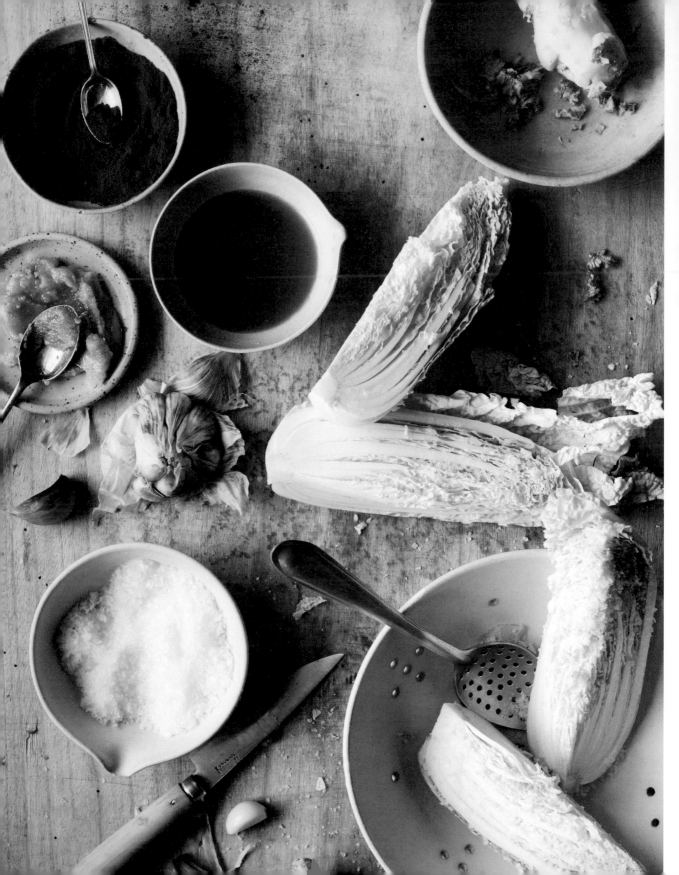

Cabbage & Kimchi Soup GF DF

SERVES 2 (easily doubled and leaves plenty of kimchi leftover, but the kimchi will keep indefinitely in the fridge).

238 cals | 7g fat | 0g saturated fat | 6.5g protein | 8.5g fibre | 33g carbs | 25g sugars | 5.8g salt

1 tbsp olive or rapeseed oil

1 small onion, finely chopped

10g dried shitake mushrooms, soaked in warm water

150g cabbage – savoy/ green pointed/hispi, finely shredded into 3cm lengths

2 tbsp miso paste

600ml freshly boiled water

1 tbsp soy sauce

150g kimchi, finely chopped (include some of the liquid)

gochugang paste (Korean chilli paste), to taste

a few drops of sesame oil

a few sprigs of coriander, finely chopped (optional)

salt and pepper

Optional extra:

a block of silken tofu, diced, or 2 eggs, poached

This is a really wholesome cabbage soup. So good for you and so tasty, too. The fermented kimchi vegetables give the broth a really deep and rich flavour. You can use shop-bought kimchi, but it's very easy to make so I've included a quick recipe for this as well (see page 256).

For the soup

Heat the oil in a saucepan and add the onion. Fry on quite a high heat – you want it to lightly caramelise rather than soften. Drain the mushrooms, reserving the soaking liquor, then add them to the onion along with the cabbage. Sauté for another 3–4 minutes.

Whisk the miso paste into the boiled water and pour over the cabbage. Season with salt and pepper and the soy sauce. Bring to the boil, then turn down, cover and simmer until the cabbage is very tender – around 10 minutes. Add the kimchi and continue to simmer for another 5 minutes.

Taste again for seasoning, heat and sweetness. Add the gochugang paste if you think it needs it and stir to dissolve.

Serve ladled into bowls with a few drops of sesame oil and some finely chopped coriander, if you like.

To make this more substantial, add protein in the form of a poached egg or tofu. For the egg, you can either break it straight into the soup and leave to simmer until the whites are just cooked through, or cook it separately. To do this, bring a saucepan of water to the boil and add 1 tbsp white vinegar. Stir the water to make a whirlpool and crack an egg into the centre – the whites will form round the yolk. Leave to simmer until you can see the whites are just cooked through, then remove with a slotted spoon and drain before dropping into the soup.

If using tofu, simply add to the soup when serving, allowing it to heat through in the broth.

A simple kimchi

1 head of Chinese cabbage

1 tbsp sea salt

spring or filtered water, for rinsing

For the paste:

4 garlic cloves, crushed

15g piece of ginger, grated

2 tbsp fish sauce

1 tsp palm sugar

1–3 tsp Kashmiri chilli powder or chilli flakes, to taste

Optional extras:

bunch of spring onions, cut into rounds

1 large carrot, shredded

1 mooli or a few radishes, shredded

coriander sprigs

micro herbs

The kimchi can be used immediately, but it's better left overnight or (even better) for two days before refrigerating and using. You don't have to use Chinese cabbage – you can use the equivalent volume in savoy cabbage, kale, spring greens or sprouts. Spring/filtered water is best for rinsing because the chlorine in tap water can inhibit fermentation.

Prepare the cabbage by cutting it into quarters lengthways and cutting into thick strips. Put in a bowl and sprinkle with the salt. Massage the salt into the cabbage until the leaves start to look wilted. Cover with a plate and weigh down with a couple of tins and leave to stand for an hour or so, until you can see that the cabbage is sitting in a pool of water. Drain off the water, then rinse thoroughly with spring or filtered water. Taste and if it is still very salty, rinse once more and drain thoroughly.

Mix all the paste ingredients together. Add any of the optional vegetables to the cabbage, then pour over the paste and mix thoroughly. Pack into a sterilised jar, making sure there are no air bubbles to be seen, then seal and leave overnight. The next day, unseal to release any gases and leave for another 24 hours. At this point the kimchi should be fermenting and can be transferred to the fridge. It will continue to ferment slowly in the fridge and will keep indefinitely.

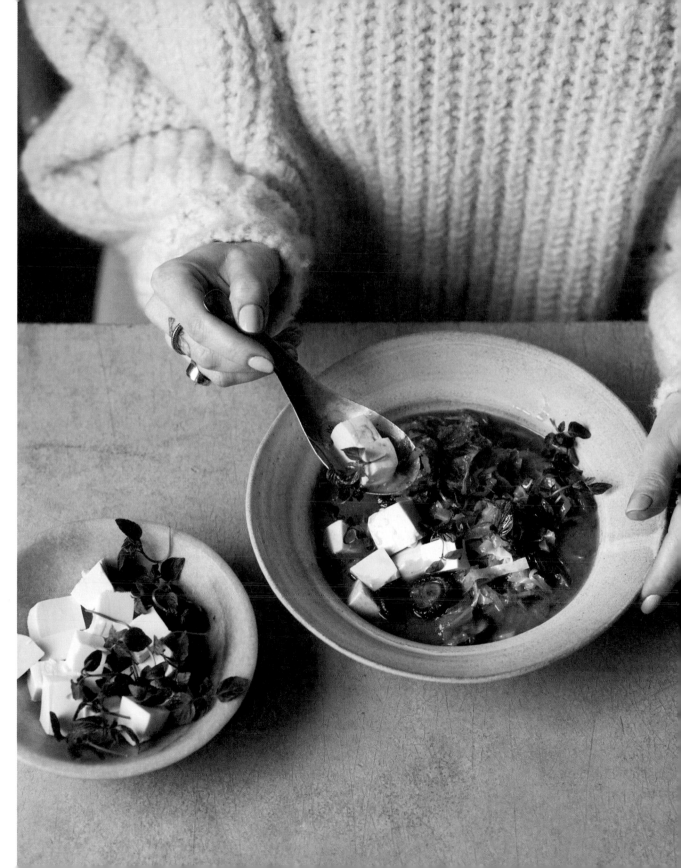

Thai Vegetable Soup GF DF

SERVES 2 generously

316 cals | 19g fat | 15g saturated fat | 1g protein | 10g fibre | 20g carbs | 14g sugars | 3.6g salt

For the paste:

2 shallots or 1 small onion, peeled and finely chopped

2–4 bird's eye red chillies (depending on how hot you like it), chopped

4 garlic cloves, roughly chopped

25g piece of ginger, roughly chopped

10g piece of turmeric, roughly chopped, or ½ tsp ground turmeric

2 lemongrass stalks, roughly chopped

zest of 1 lime

6 lime leaves

For the broth:

500ml vegetable stock

200ml coconut milk

1–2 tbsp fish sauce

juice of 1 lime

½ tsp palm or coconut sugar (optional)

salt

I'm a big fan of spice – especially these delicious Thai flavours. I love this at the end of the day when I've had a busy week with work. It's similar in style to a light and lean Tom Yum soup. The recipe below makes more paste than you need for two portions of soup, but it will store in the fridge for a week, or freezes very well too, so is worth doing. Alternatively, a shop-bought Thai red-curry paste can be used. As for vegetables, anything goes, especially whatever is in season – you could use cabbage, kale, pak choi, squash or pumpkin, mooli or pea aubergines.

First make the paste. Put everything in a small food processor or blender and pulse, pushing down the sides regularly until it forms a paste. The texture won't be completely smooth, but you don't want it very coarse either – try to make sure everything is finely chopped. You might find adding a tablespoon or two of water will help.

To make the broth, put the vegetable stock and coconut milk into a saucepan. Add half the paste and bring to the boil. Turn down to a simmer and add 1 tablespoon of the fish sauce and the lime juice and sugar, if using. Stir to combine and start to add the vegetables – add the carrot, red pepper and baby corn. Bring to the boil, then turn down and simmer for 5 minutes, then add the courgette and broccoli spears or asparagus tips. Simmer until all the vegetables are tender, then add the beansprouts and spring onions.

Taste for seasoning and add more of the paste, fish sauce or salt if necessary. Add any of the optional extras, then garnish with the herbs. Serve with chilli oil on the side and lime wedges for squeezing.

For the vegetables:

1 carrot, cut into thin slices

½ red pepper, sliced lengthways

6 baby corn, cut into chunks

1 courgette, cut into ribbons

6 sprouting broccoli spears or 8 asparagus tips, halved lengthways

handful of beansprouts

4 spring onions, cut in half lengthways and finely shredded (no larger than 1mm)

Optional extras:

1 block of silken tofu (200–250g), drained and diced

150g prawns, cooked

100g brown or wild rice, cooked

To serve:

small bunches of Thai basil and/or coriander and mint

chilli oil

lime wedges

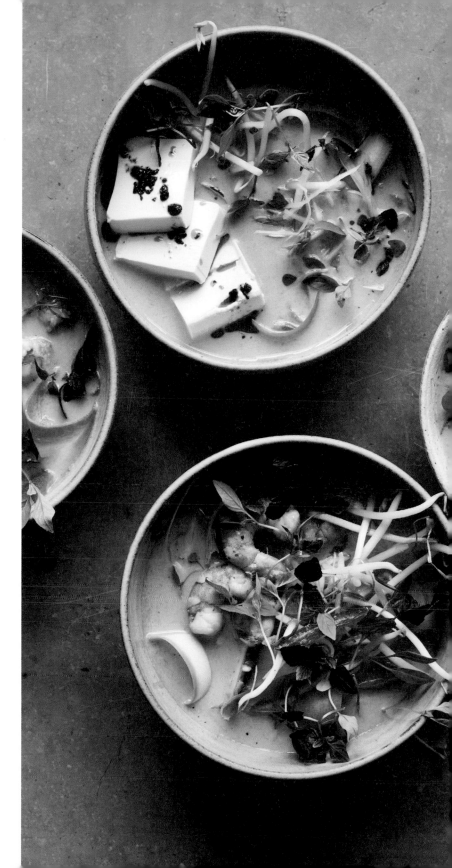

MAINS

Stir-fries

SERVES 2

Oil:

2 tbsp vegetable or groundnut oil

Choose at least one from each of these categories (if you're stuck for ideas, you'll find a delicious selection overleaf):

Protein (optional)

Aromatics – all finely chopped or grated

Vegetables – all sliced uniformly

Tender greens – all shredded/thinly sliced

Additional low/no-cook vegetables that just need heating through

Sauce:

2 tbsp soy sauce, tamari or fish sauce, as a base

Plus any sauces from the selection overleaf

Stir-fries are my go-to midweek dinners – easy, quick and delicious. I try to use lots of fresh vegetables, aromatics and spices rather than processed sauces, as they tend to have a long list of ingredients and additives, including tons of sugar. Use as many components as you like from the lists that follow – there are so many tasty variations. Turn the page for some of my favourite options.

My top tip is to make sure everything is prepped and ready to go before you start cooking.

First, cook any carbohydrates you might want to add – cook noodles or rice according to the packet instructions and leave to cool. Toss noodles in a little sesame oil to stop them sticking.

Make a sauce. Soy, fish sauce or tamari are good bases to start with, then add in any of the other flavours from the list on the following page and set aside.

Make sure any vegetables and garnishes are prepped and ready to add when you need them.

If adding protein, add seasoning and lightly dust in cornflour before cooking. Heat 1 tablespoon oil in a wok. When the air is shimmering above the oil, add the protein and stir-fry until crisp and lightly browned, then remove. If using egg, use just 1 teaspoon oil, add the egg and let it coat the base of the wok. When it is just set, break it up into strips and remove.

Carb element:

Noodles or rice (my suggestions can be found on the following pages)

Garnishes:

Any of the garnishes listed overleaf

Wipe out the wok and add the remaining oil. Add any aromatics – garlic, ginger, etc. – and stir-fry for a minute, followed by at least three of the firmer vegetables. Stir-fry these for another couple of minutes, then add at least one green. Continue stir-frying for 2–3 minutes, then pour in the sauce. Simmer for another 2–3 minutes, then add at least one from the final group of vegetables. Return any protein to the wok and add any carbohydrates.

Add any garnishes and divide between two bowls.

LOW-CARB STIR-FRY: Cook prawns or extra firm tofu as above. Add ginger, garlic, lemongrass and lime leaves, then shallots, baby corn, asparagus, sprouting broccoli and beansprouts. Make a sauce using fish sauce, lime juice, hot sauce, add back the prawns or tofu and garnish with spring onions, pumpkin seeds, coriander, mint or Thai basil.

BROWN RICE STIR-FRY: Cook 1 egg as above. Fry ginger and garlic, then carrot, red pepper, hispi cabbage and peas. Make a sauce from soy sauce, rice vinegar, rice wine and Chinese five spice. Add 100g cooked brown rice, garnish with coriander, sesame oil and seeds.

CHOOSE YOUR CARB:

75g uncooked glass noodles or soba (buckwheat) noodles

100g cooked brown rice

CHOOSE YOUR SAUCE FLAVOURINGS:

Add any of:

1 tbsp rice wine, mirin or Shaoxing wine

1 tbsp rice wine vinegar or citrus juice (yuzu, lime, lemon, mandarin)

1 tsp hot sauce or gochugang paste

1 tsp curry powder or ½ tsp Chinese five-spice powder

½ tsp palm or coconut sugar

PICK YOUR PROTEIN:

Lightly coated in cornflour or rice flour:

150g prawns, fish goujons, squid, extra-firm tofu or tempeh

Or

2 tbsp nuts (cashew or peanuts) or 1 egg, beaten

THE AROMATICS:

All finely chopped or grated:

15g piece of ginger

2 garlic cloves

1 lemongrass stalk

2 lime leaves

5g piece of turmeric

2 tbsp kimchi (see page 256)

1 tbsp fermented black beans

MAKE YOUR OWN STIR-FRY

THE VEGETABLES:

|

Firmer veg – at least three of the following, all sliced uniformly:

2 shallots or 1 small red/white onion

1 pepper

100g baby corn

1 large carrot

6 radishes

100g mushrooms

150g cauliflower florets, broccoli florets, Romanesco or sprouting broccoli

100g green beans, asparagus, mangetout or sugar snap peas

150g any type of cabbage, Brussels sprouts or spring greens

|

Tender greens – at least one of the following, all shredded/thinly sliced:

100g spinach

200g kale or chard leaves

200g pak choi or similar, or courgette

|

Low or no-cook vegetables that just need heating through – choose at least one:

50g peas, sweetcorn, beansprouts or bamboo shoots

50g water chestnuts, sliced

FINALLY, CHOOSE YOUR GARNISH:

Any of the below:

|

2 spring onions, either cut into rounds or halved lengthways and shredded

handfuls of coriander, mint, Thai basil

sesame oil and/or 1 tsp sesame seeds

1 tbsp pumpkin seeds

Fish Tacos GF DF

SERVES 2

781 cals | 28g fat | 5g saturated fat | 42g protein | 14g fibre | 83g carbs | 12g sugars | 2g salt

For the fish:

all but ½ tsp of the spice mix
(see below)

1 tbsp olive oil

1 tsp chipotle paste

zest of 1 lime

2 skinned fillets of fish,
cut into cubes

For the spice mix:

1 tsp ground cumin

½ tsp dried oregano

½ tsp garlic powder

¼ tsp ground cinnamon

¼ tsp allspice

salt

**For the black bean and
orange salsa:**

1 orange (see method and tip
opposite)

½ red onion, finely sliced

juice of 1 lime

100g black beans, rinsed

1 garlic clove, finely chopped

1 jalapeño, finely chopped

½ tsp of the spice mix (see
above)

1 tsp red wine vinegar

small bunch of coriander

There are lots of components to this recipe, but it is actually very quick and easy to assemble – and it never fails to impress my friends. I love the zestiness of the lime with the fish. The key to success with the salsa is to chop everything as finely as you can.

First marinade the fish. Make the spice mix by mixing everything together and seasoning with salt, then put all but ½ a teaspoon into a bowl. Mix with the olive oil, chipotle paste and lime zest and add a little water. Add the fish and toss very gently (you don't want it to break up) until completely coated. Cover and leave to marinate in the fridge for at least an hour.

Next make the salsa. Prepare the orange by topping and tailing it, cutting away the pith and dicing the flesh (see tip opposite). Put it into a bowl and squeeze any juice from the discarded orange peel over it. Put the red onion in a separate bowl and sprinkle with salt. Pour over the lime juice and leave to stand for 30 minutes. Mix all the other ingredients with the orange and add the onion just before serving – it should be a bright pink.

For the avocado, put the lime juice in a small bowl with a large pinch of salt and add the avocado. Mash until smooth.

When you are ready to assemble, heat up the tortillas. Do this by warming a dry frying pan over a medium heat. Heat the tortillas one by one – they should just need around 15 seconds on each side. Keep them warm by wrapping in a tea towel.

For the avocado:

juice of 1 lime

1 avocado, diced

To serve:

6–8 small corn tortillas, depending how hungry you are

2 spring onions, halved and shredded lengthways

1 Little Gem lettuce or similar, shredded

a few sprigs of coriander

lime wedges

To fry the fish, heat 1 tablespoon olive oil in a frying pan. Fry the pieces of fish until cooked through and browned on all sides.

To serve, arrange everything on the table for self assembly.

TIP: *How to segment an orange.* Top and tail, then, following along the curve of the orange, cut away the skin and outer membrane. Trim off any remaining pith. Holding the orange in your hand over a bowl to catch any juice, cut the segments out as close to the membrane as you can. Squeeze juice from the membrane before discarding. Use the juice in the salad dressing.

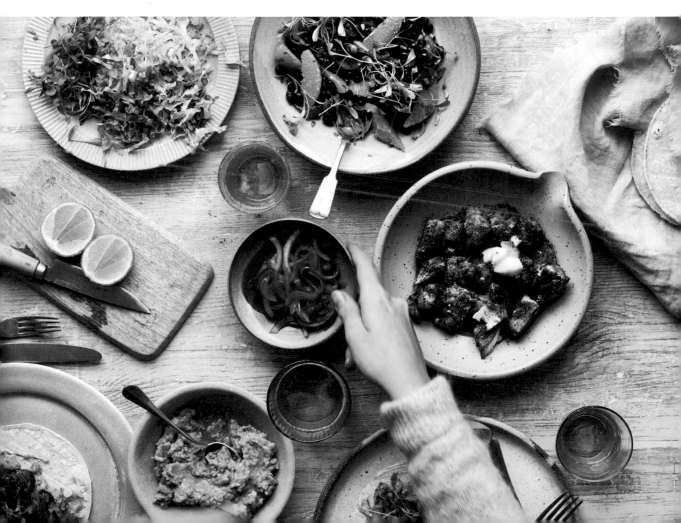

Roast Vegetable & Fish Traybake

  SERVES 2

655 cals | 32g fat | 5.5g saturated fat | 40g protein | 16.5g fibre | 36g carbs | 12g sugars | 1.4g salt

1 red onion, cut into wedges

1 red or green pepper, deseeded and cut into thick strips

1 courgette, cut into 1cm slices on the diagonal

1 fennel bulb, trimmed and cut into wedges (optional)

2 tbsp olive oil

1 tsp dried thyme or oregano

100ml white wine or water

1 x 400g tin cannellini beans, drained (optional)

8 cherry tomatoes

salt and pepper

For the fish:

2 skinned fish fillets (sea bass, bream or thicker fillets of cod/similar)

25g pitted olives

25g capers

zest of 1 lemon

handful of basil leaves

15g nibbed pistachios or flaked almonds

3 slices of lemon

To serve:

basil leaves or parsley

This is my take on a Sunday roast, although it's so easy to make you can also have it midweek when you get home from work – it all cooks in one roasting tin, too, so leaves you with a lot less washing up! I make this with all sorts of different vegetables, so it's a great dish for using up leftovers as well. Don't scrimp on the herbs – these make all the difference.

Preheat the oven to 200°C. Put the vegetables in a large roasting tin and drizzle over the olive oil. Sprinkle with the thyme or oregano and season with salt and pepper. Roast in the oven for 35–40 minutes, stirring halfway through, until the vegetables are tender and slightly browned around the edges.

While the vegetables are roasting, prepare the fish. Season the fillets with salt and pepper. Put the olives, capers, lemon zest, basil leaves and pistachios or almonds into a food processor or blender and pulse until you have a coarse paste. Spread the paste over one side of the fish fillets. Top each with a slice of lemon.

Remove the roasting tin from the oven. Pour the wine or water around the vegetables and add the cannellini beans, if using, and cherry tomatoes.

Arrange the fish fillets over the vegetables and roast for another 10–15 minutes, depending on how thick the fish is.

Remove from the oven and divide between two warmed plates. Sprinkle over some roughly torn basil leaves and serve with lemon wedges.

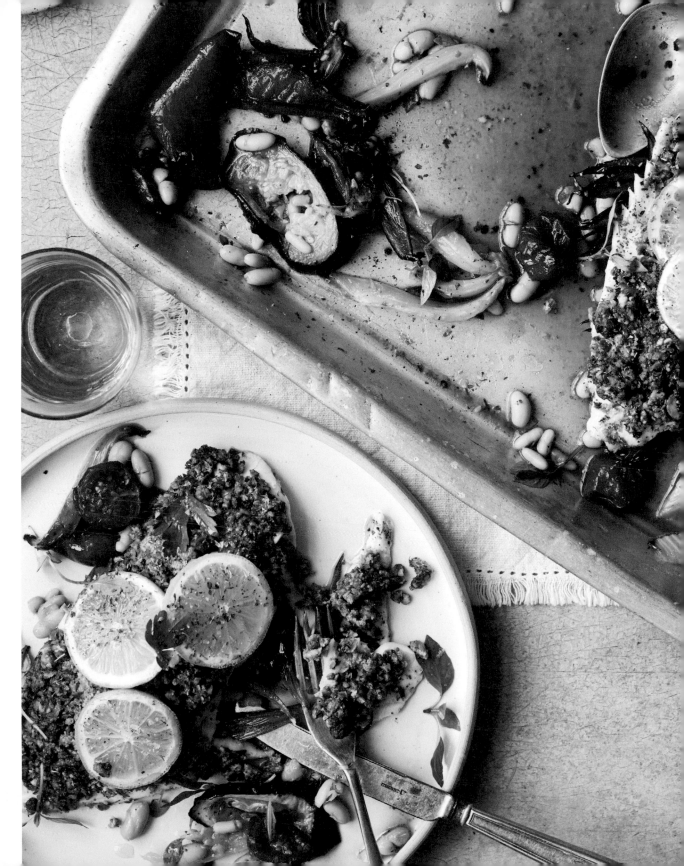

Aubergine Balls with Tomato Sauce

   SERVES 2

420 cals | 23g fat | 3g saturated fat | 9g protein | 10.5g fibre | 30g carbs | 15g sugars | 0.6g salt

For the aubergine balls:

2 tbsp olive oil, plus extra for brushing

1 small onion, finely chopped

1 large aubergine (around 300g), finely diced

2 garlic cloves, finely chopped

1 tsp dried oregano

small bunch of flat-leaf parsley, finely chopped

zest of 1 lemon

100g well-cooked brown rice, roughly puréed

25g milled flax seeds

salt and pepper

For the tomato sauce:

1 tbsp olive oil

1 small onion, finely chopped

2 garlic cloves, finely chopped

1 tsp dried oregano

a pinch of ground cinnamon

100ml red wine

1 x 400g tin chopped tomatoes

a few basil leaves

If you like meatballs but want to go easy on meat, you'll love these. I've used flax seed to bind these instead of egg, in order to make the recipe vegan, but you can adapt this if you want. They work great with gluten-free pasta, a pile of greens or a fresh green salad.

First make the aubergine balls. Heat the olive oil in a frying pan and add the onion and aubergine. Fry on a low heat to start with, until the onion is starting to look translucent and the aubergine is softening, then turn up the heat and continue to cook, stirring regularly, until they are lightly caramelised. Make sure the aubergine is completely cooked through, then add the garlic and cook for a further 2 minutes.

Preheat the oven to 200°C.

Transfer to a bowl to cool, then stir in the oregano, parsley, lemon zest, brown rice and flax seeds. Season with salt and pepper. Mix thoroughly – it should clump together easily – then form into eight balls.

Arrange on a baking tray and brush with olive oil. Bake in the oven for 20 minutes, turning over once.

To make the sauce, heat the olive oil in a saucepan and add the onion. Sauté until the onion is soft and translucent, then add the garlic and cook for another couple of minutes. Add the oregano and cinnamon, then pour in the red wine. Bring to the boil and keep boiling until the wine has reduced by half. Add the tomatoes and season with salt and pepper.

Return to the boil, then turn down the heat, cover and simmer for 20 minutes.

When the aubergine balls are baked, remove from the oven. Transfer the tomato sauce to a shallow pan and stir in a few basil leaves. Add the aubergine balls and simmer for a few minutes to let the aubergines take on some flavour from the sauce. Serve with plenty of greens.

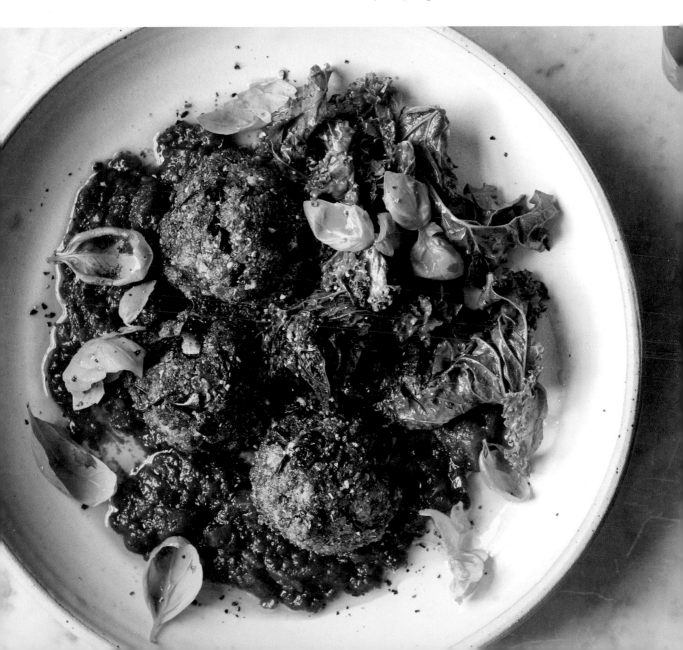

Shepherd's Pie (VN) (GF) (DF)

SERVES 4

514 cals | 12g fat | 2g saturated fat | 16g protein | 21g fibre | 66g carbs | 15.5g sugars | 0.6g salt

1 tbsp olive oil

1 onion, finely chopped

1 stick celery, finely chopped

1 large carrot, finely diced

2 garlic cloves, finely chopped

1 sprig of rosemary, finely chopped

2 bay leaves

200g cooked lentils (Puy or brown)

100ml red wine

1 tsp Dijon mustard

1 tbsp tomato purée

dash of Worcestershire sauce or mushroom ketchup

100g broad beans (frozen work well)

300g peas

100g kale, chopped

400ml vegetable stock or water

salt and pepper

For the mash:

400g sweet potatoes, peeled and diced

400g celeriac, peeled and diced

75ml plant-based milk

2 tbsp olive oil

This is the ultimate comfort meal – perfect for those nights when you just want to stay home and hibernate. With the veggie filling and sweet potato and celeriac topping, this is a healthy twist on a classic shepherd's pie, but just as delicious and warming.

This recipe will be enough for a round ovenproof dish of around 24cm diameter.

Heat the olive oil in a lidded frying pan and add the onion, celery and carrot. Sauté on a medium heat until the vegetables are starting to soften and are lightly caramelised around the edges. Add the garlic and herbs and cook for a further couple of minutes.

Stir in the lentils, then pour over the red wine. Bring to the boil and simmer for 5 minutes. Stir in the mustard and tomato purée until they have completely dissolved into the wine, then add the Worcestershire sauce or mushroom ketchup. Season with salt and pepper.

Add the remaining vegetables and pour in the stock. Bring to the boil, then turn down the heat, cover and simmer for around 20 minutes until the vegetables are completely tender. The peas should be very soft and sweet and will have lost their bright green – this is how they are supposed to look! Simmer for a few more minutes until the sauce has reduced.

While the filling is simmering, make the mash. Bring a large pan of water to the boil and add the sweet potatoes, celeriac and plenty of salt. Simmer until they are knife tender, then drain thoroughly. Return to the saucepan and leave to steam in their own heat, covered, for another 5 minutes – this helps dry them out. Add the plant-based milk and half the olive oil and mash thoroughly. Taste for seasoning and add more salt and some pepper if necessary.

Preheat the oven to 200°C.

Pour the filling into an ovenproof dish and cover with the mash, spreading evenly with a spatula. Rough up the surface with a fork and drizzle over the remaining oil. Bake in the oven for around 30 minutes or until the top has lightly coloured.

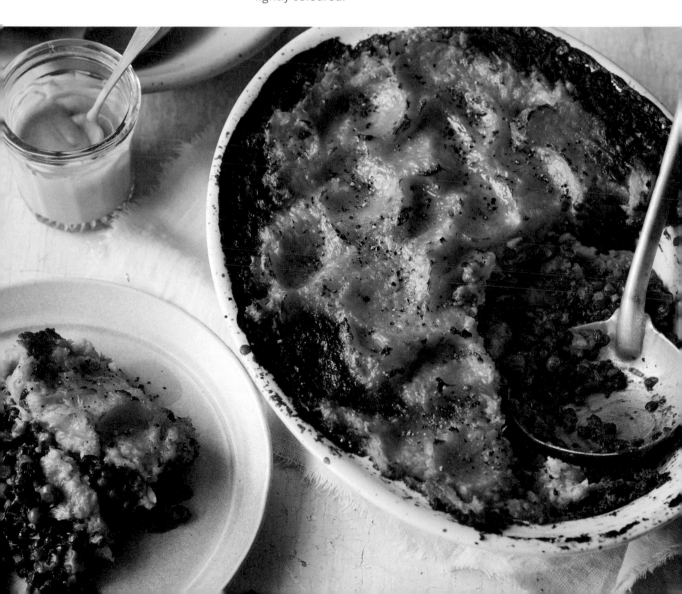

Vegetable Curry VN GF DF

SERVES 2 generously

503 cals | 27g fat | 20g saturated fat | 18g protein | 18g fibre | 38g carbs | 22g sugars | 0.3g salt

1 tbsp coconut oil

1 onion, finely chopped

1 tsp mustard seeds

1 tsp cumin seeds

3 garlic cloves, finely chopped

25g piece of ginger, finely chopped

2 tbsp coriander stems, finely chopped

½ tsp each of: ground cinnamon, ground turmeric, ground cardamom, ground coriander, ground fenugreek, cayenne pepper

2 bay leaves

100g squash or pumpkin, diced

½ red pepper, deseeded and diced

1 x 400g tin chickpeas

200ml coconut milk

200g fresh or tinned tomatoes, puréed

1 courgette, sliced

200g green beans, sprouting broccoli or okra, trimmed

100g spinach

salt and pepper

To serve:

coriander leaves or micro herbs

I love curries. A lot of people think you need to have meat in a curry, but this veggie one really hits the spot and is filling and tasty. The vegetables listed below are intended as a guide and can be varied according to what is to hand or in season – wedges of cabbage, Brussels sprouts, sweet potato and other root vegetables all work really nicely. Use the quantities here as a guide.

Heat the coconut oil in a saucepan or casserole and add the onion. Sauté on a medium heat until the onion is lightly golden, then add the mustard and cumin seeds, garlic, ginger, coriander stems, spices and bay leaves. Cook for a couple of minutes until the onion looks well coated, then add the squash and red pepper.

Season with salt and pepper, then pour in 150ml water. Bring to the boil, then cover and simmer for 5 minutes. Add the chickpeas, coconut milk and tomatoes and bring to the boil again. Simmer for another 5 minutes, then add the courgette and beans, sprouting broccoli or okra, leaving them on top so they'll steam. Cover and simmer until the vegetables are tender – around another 20 minutes – checking regularly and adding a splash of water if necessary. Stir in the spinach and wait for it to wilt down.

To make the cauliflower rice, pulse the cauliflower in a food processor or blender, or finely chop it so it resembles coarse breadcrumbs. Add the nigella seeds, if using, to a dry frying pan and toast for a few minutes until they have a strong aroma. Pour around 50ml water in the pan and add the cauliflower. Season with salt and pepper and cook on a

For the cauliflower rice:

½ cauliflower, broken up into florets

1 tsp nigella seeds (optional)

medium heat for around 5 minutes, stirring regularly, until all the water has evaporated and the cauliflower is dry and more translucent in appearance.

Serve the curry with the cauliflower rice, garnished with coriander and lemon wedges on the side.

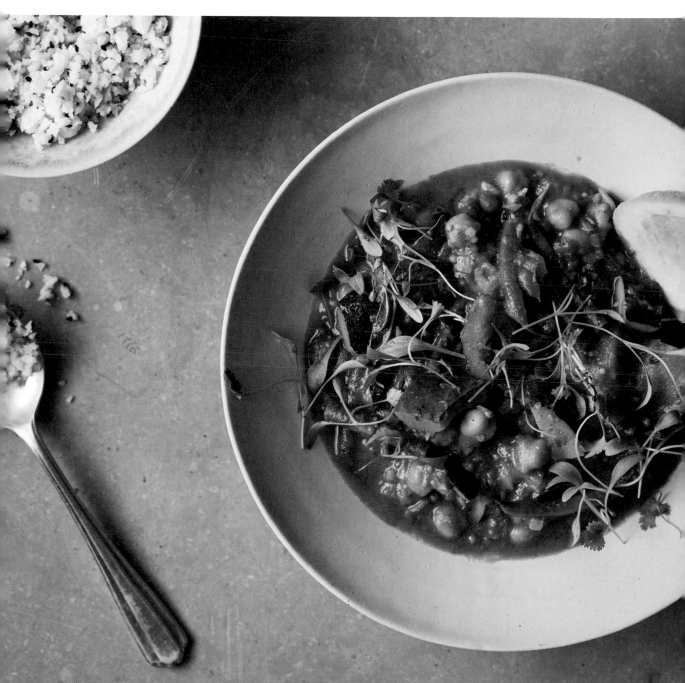

SWEET STUFF

Blueberry & Peach Crumble

SERVES 2–3

693 cals | 44g fat | 12g saturated fat | 16g protein | 4g fibre | 57g carbs | 34g sugars | 0.1g salt

For the base:

1 ripe peach or nectarine, pitted and cut into wedges

100g blueberries

1 tbsp maple syrup, honey or coconut sugar

juice of ½ lemon

1 tbsp cornflour or arrowroot

For the topping:

60g ground almonds

40g flaked almonds

1 tbsp flax seeds

1 tbsp coconut sugar

2 tbsp coconut oil

For the custard:

250ml plant-based milk (I used almond to complement the pudding)

½ tsp vanilla extract

1 tbsp maple syrup or coconut sugar (or your choice of sweetener)

2 tbsp cornflour or custard powder (preferably custard powder)

This is a healthy twist on one of my favourite childhood desserts. The fruit used in it is pretty interchangeable: it just needs to be ripe. Generally, I go for whatever is in season, but I also keep bags of frozen fruit in the freezer. Any fresh or frozen berries will work here, mixed with any orchard fruit – apples, pears, plums, peaches or nectarines. Almond milk works really well in the custard. For the distinctive yellow colour, it is best to use custard powder – it's vegan.

Preheat the oven to 180°C.

Put the fruit into a bowl and sprinkle over your choice of sweetener, the lemon juice and the cornflour or arrowroot. Stir until the cornflour or arrowroot has completely dissolved, then transfer to a small ovenproof dish (about 12 x 18cm).

Mix all the topping ingredients together until they start clumping together, then sprinkle evenly over the fruit. Place the dish on a baking tray and bake in the oven for 30–35 minutes until golden brown and the fruit is bubbling up.

While the crumble is baking, make the custard. Put 200ml of the milk into a saucepan with the vanilla extract and maple syrup and heat gently. Mix the remaining milk with the cornflour or custard powder until you have a smooth paste. Pour this into the saucepan and continue to cook on a slightly higher heat, stirring constantly. The mixture should thicken to a custard consistency as it comes up to the boil. Make sure you stir constantly as this can happen very quickly and form a thick layer on the base of the saucepan.

Serve the crumble with custard poured over.

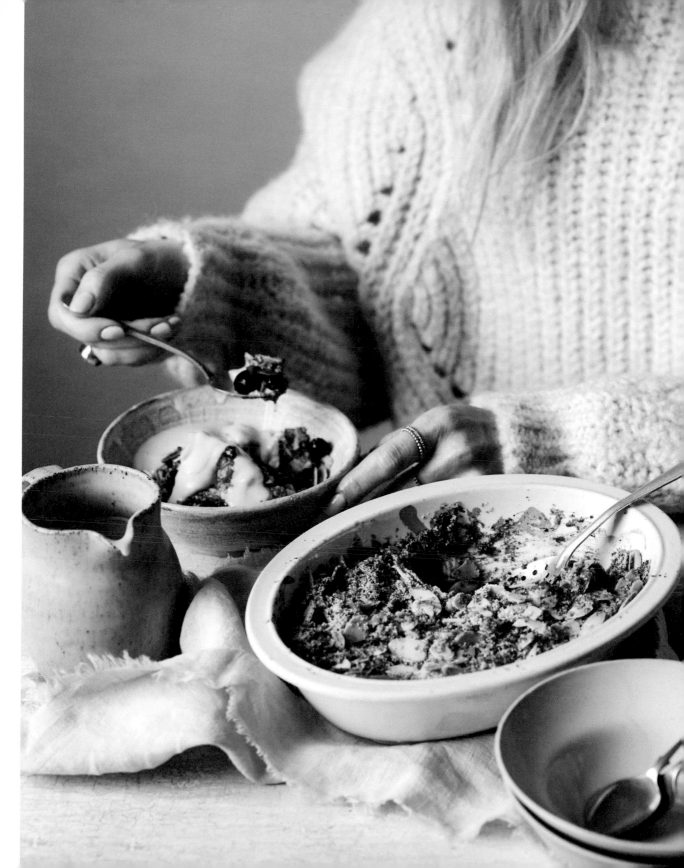

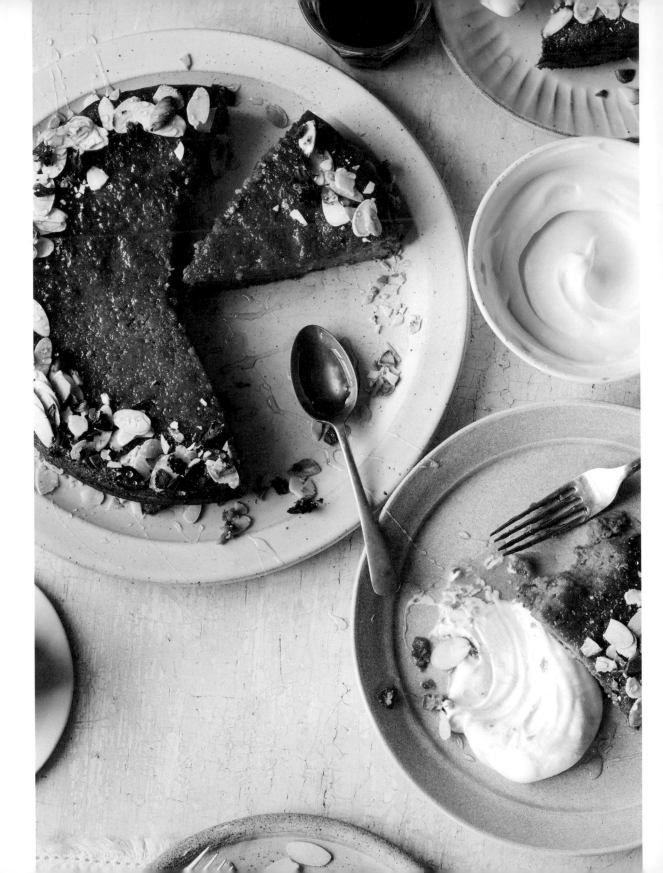

Orange & Almond Cake

MAKES 8 slices

593 cals | 46g fat | 9g saturated fat | 11g protein | 2g fibre | 34g carbs | 26g sugars | 0.6g salt

1 small orange (about 200g)

3 large eggs

100g coconut sugar

125g ground almonds

1 tsp baking powder

salt

To top:

1 tsp honey

1 tbsp orange juice

1 tbsp flaked almonds, toasted (optional)

1 tsp dried rose petals (optional)

To serve (optional):

100ml plant-based double cream

1 tsp honey

I don't believe in depriving yourself of the foods you love, so it was really important to me to include some healthier sweet treats. This delicious cake is so sweet and full of flavour, but it doesn't use any white refined sugar. The orange, almond and honey work together perfectly.

Put the orange in a saucepan of water and bring to the boil. Simmer until the orange is very soft – the best way to tell is to push the handle of a wooden spoon through the skin – if it pierces it easily, the orange will be done. This will take at least an hour, but can be done in advance.

When the orange is cool enough to handle, break it open and remove any seeds and the central core of white pith. Put the rest of the orange into a food processor or blender and blitz to a purée.

Preheat the oven to 170°C and line an 18cm round tin with baking parchment.

Put the eggs in a bowl with a pinch of salt and whisk until they are very aerated and frothy – they will still be very liquid. Whisk in the coconut sugar, followed by the ground almonds and the baking powder, then fold in the orange. Pour into the prepared tin and bake for 35–40 minutes until lightly browned, springy to touch and shrinking away from the sides.

Melt the honey and orange juice together, then use to brush the top of the warm cake. Sprinkle with the toasted almonds and rose petals, if using.

If serving with the cream, put into a bowl with the honey and whisk until it forms soft peaks. The cake will keep for up to a week in an airtight tin.

Chocolate Mousse

MAKES 2 generous portions, or 4 small

228 cals | 11g fat | 6g saturated fat | 2g protein | 1g fibre | 31g carbs | 29g sugars | 0.6g salt

75ml aquafaba (liquid from a tin of unsalted chickpeas)

75g raw chocolate (I used a 85% cocoa-solids bar made with coconut sugar)

15ml maple syrup

25ml almond milk

½ tsp vanilla extract

a generous pinch each of chilli powder, ground cinnamon and ground ginger

salt

Your choice of toppings:

cacao nibs

pistachios

goji berries

This is my ultimate comfort pudding. I have made it as nutritious as possible using raw chocolate and coconut sugar, but it tastes as delicious as any mousse I've tried. The whisked aquafaba keeps this recipe so light and airy (just make sure you definitely use liquid from an unsalted tin of chickpeas). I love mine with cacao nibs sprinkled on top, which add a nice crunchy texture and also give you a great burst of energy.

First whisk the aquafaba – the easiest way to do this is in a stand mixer as it does take time; otherwise use electric beaters. Whisk until it reaches the stiff-peak stage – it should look dry and glossy.

While the aquafaba is mixing, melt the raw chocolate by placing it in a heatproof bowl over a saucepan of simmering water. When it has melted, remove from the heat and add the remaining ingredients along with a small pinch of salt. Whisk thoroughly until you have a smooth dark liquid.

Mix a heaped tablespoon of the aquafaba into the chocolate mix to loosen it, then add the rest, stirring lightly but thoroughly to keep the volume but making sure there are no streaks. Divide between two large or four small glasses or ramekins and transfer to the fridge. Leave for a couple of hours to chill and firm up.

Serve with your choice of garnishes.

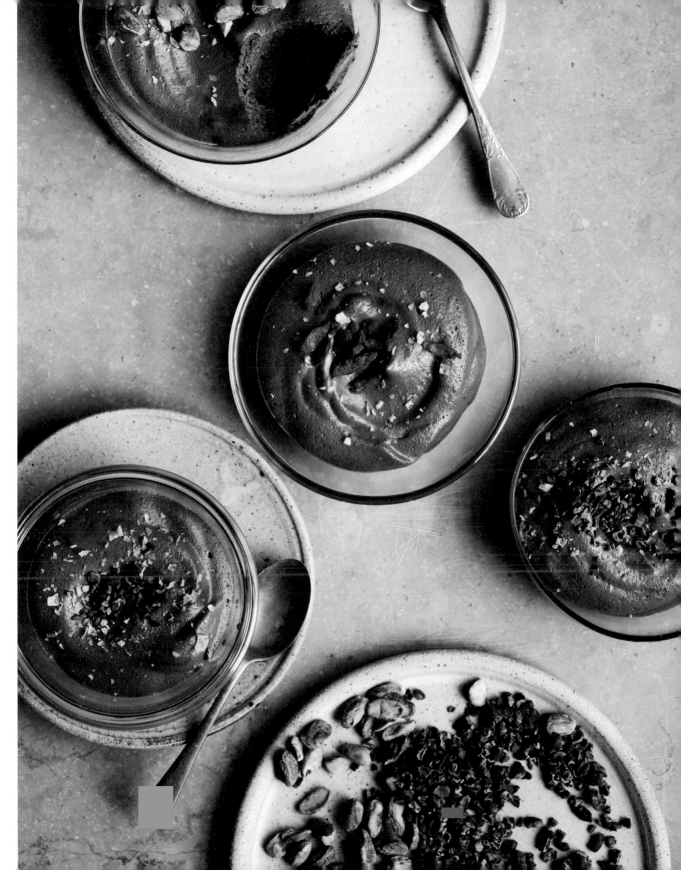

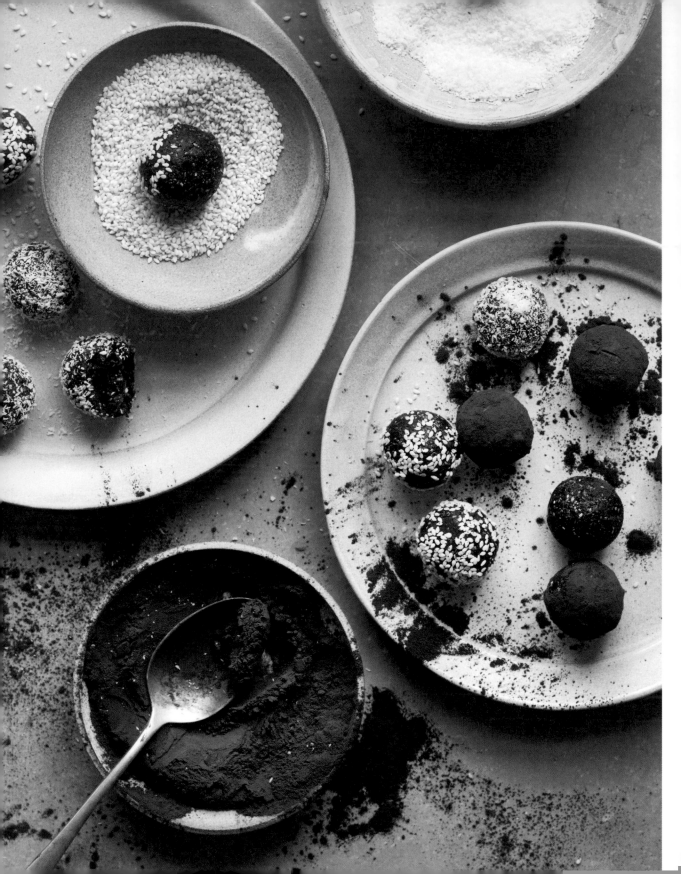

Energy Balls

MAKES 16

96 cals | 6g fat | 2g saturated fat | 3g protein | 3g fibre | 6g carbs | 5g sugars | 0.1g salt

150g dried fruit – pitted dates, figs, pitted prunes, apricots

75g nut butter (any sort)

1 tbsp honey

2 tbsp cacao powder (optional)

25g desiccated coconut or coconut flour

25g finely chopped nuts (Brazil nuts are good)

25g flax seeds

25g chia seeds

salt

To coat (optional):

1 tbsp cacao powder or similar, OR 2 tbsp desiccated coconut or sesame seeds

These little energy balls are a great pick-me-up. I make them in big batches and often grab one or two when I'm on the go, or those times when a hectic schedule means I have to wait a bit longer between meals. They can be made with any of the large dried fruits – dates, figs, prunes, apricots. The only thing to remember is that if you aren't using the very soft, ready-to-eat sort, they will need soaking first.

If using dried as opposed to the ready-to-eat, softened dried fruits, soak them in warm water for 30 minutes. Drain and chop as finely as you can – roughly chopping and putting in a food processor or blender will also work. Mix in all the remaining ingredients along with a large pinch of salt. Mix thoroughly with your hands. The mixture will feel dry and crumbly to start with but will eventually come together into one sticky mass. Divide into sixteen small balls.

If you want to roll the balls in a coating, put them in the fridge to chill first.

Store in the fridge: they will keep for several weeks.

VARIATIONS: Matching fruit with nuts works well, e.g. apricots with pistachios. Spices can be added in – ground cinnamon, ground ginger, chilli powder – in addition to or in place of the cacao. The cacao can be replaced with other powders – e.g. maca, baobab, lacuma – but in smaller quantities (a teaspoon each).

Customised Raw Chocolate Bars

  VN GF DF

MAKES one 18 x 24cm bar

(Alternatively, individual bars can be made in silicone moulds or cupcake cases.)

129 cals | 9.5g fat | 5g saturated fat | 2g protein | 1g fibre | 8g carbs | 7g sugars | 0g salt

100g cacao butter or coconut oil or butter, melted

60g cacao powder

80ml liquid sweetener e.g. maple syrup

a few drops of vanilla extract

Add any of the following:

sweet spices (cardamom, cinnamon, nutmeg, ginger, chilli, black pepper), citrus zest (orange, lime)

For sprinkling:

2 tbsp finely chopped or nibbed nuts, 2 tbsp finely chopped dried fruit, 2 tbsp goji berries, 2 tbsp finely chopped crystallised ginger or citrus peel

I love chocolate as much as the next person, but these customised raw chocolate bars are so much better than anything you can buy in the shops. This recipe sets really well and the texture is very smooth. I like to add goji berries, which are delicious and so good for you. You could also add nibbed pistachios and a bit of crystallised ginger on top and include pinches of ground cardamom, cinnamon and black pepper in the base. There are so many possibilities once you start experimenting.

A few things to remember: if you make them with coconut oil they will need to be stored in the fridge. Cacao butter/coconut butter gives a better set for storing at room temperature.

Melt the cacao butter, coconut oil or coconut butter, then pour into a bowl. Add the cacao powder, sweetener, a few drops of vanilla extract and any spices you might want to use (a generous pinch to start with and taste: you can always add more).

Line a small dish with baking parchment and pour the chocolatey mixture onto it in an even layer. Sprinkle with your choice of fruits and nuts.

Leave in the fridge until set solid. Leave whole and break off as you want it, or cut into shards with a sharp knife.

Store in an airtight container; in the fridge if using coconut oil; or in the fridge or at room temperature if using the cacao butter or coconut butter.

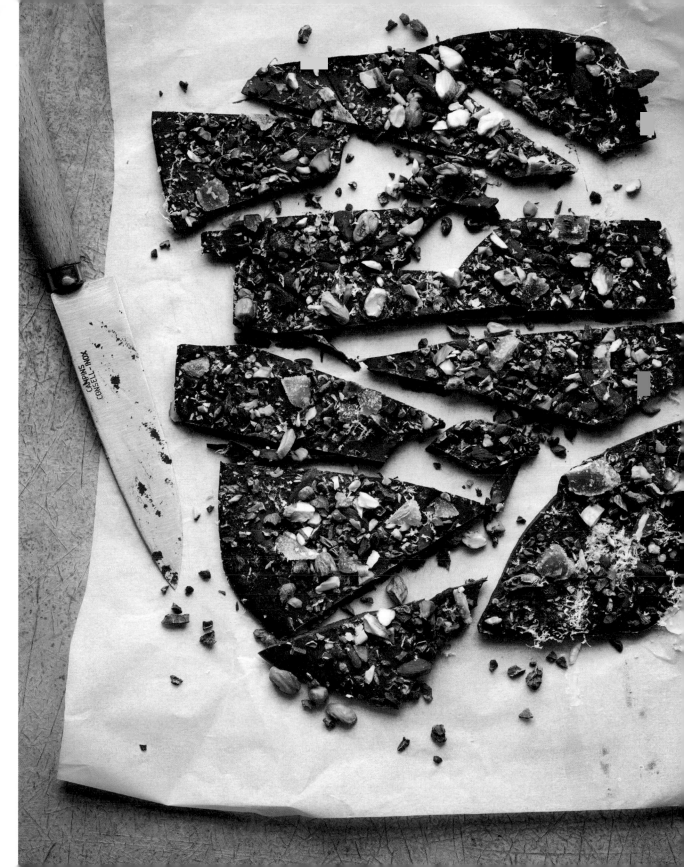

RECIPE INDEX

First published in Great Britain in 2021 by Seven Dials
an imprint of The Orion Publishing Group Ltd
Carmelite House, 50 Victoria Embankment
London EC4Y 0DZ

An Hachette UK Company

10 9 8 7 6 5 4 3 2 1

Publisher: Vicky Eribo
Project editor: Ru Merritt
Recipe development: Catherine Phipps
Art direction and design: Helen Ewing
Cover design: Smith & Gilmour
Production: Claire Keep
Photography: Issy Croker
Food styling: Emily Ezekiel
Clothes styling: Nathan Klein
Make-up: Lucy Wearing
Hair: Nick Latham at The Hair Bros
Photography (boxing imagery): Jennifer McCord, Andrew Timms
Artist management: TaP Management

A CIP catalogue record for this book is
available from the British Library.

ISBN (Hardback) 978 1 8418 8506 3
ISBN (eBook) 978 1 8418 8507 0

Printed in Italy

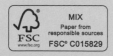

www.orionbooks.co.uk